LOVE IN THE PRISON
OF PSYCHOSIS

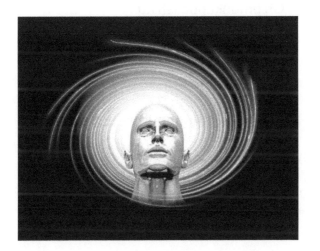

By Nick Clark

'One million people commit suicide every year.'
The World Health Organization

Nick Clark

Published by
Chipmunkapublishing
PO Box 6872
Brentwood
Essex CM13 1ZT
United Kingdom

http://www.chipmunkapublishing.com

Proof-read by Anna Gomez

LOVE IN THE PRISON OF PSYCHOSIS

Where does one start?

Right now…it is 10:39am on Monday 17th October 2005. Space and time. Do I start to spin a memory? Or do I tell my dreams? Do I explain in detail the prison I am in? Or do I try to create a fiction from the wealth of ideas that are my best comfort? What series of words will create the necessary structure by which you will see in my paragraphs that which I might want you to perceive? Will I say it all wrongly? Will my diatribe flow forth from my brain like a waterfall of potent data, or will my scribing be the lacklustre efforts of a poisoned mind caught in a monumental decay? Will the entity that is 'Nick Clark' never be allowed to produce his thoughts officially, as he remains locked into a spiral of psychosis that causes his brain fluctuations to waver on the cusp of horror? Will this unceasing tirade of auditory and visual hallucination never remedy itself, allowing me to return back to 'normality' – whatever that may be?

What I really want to do is tell the truth. But I don't know what the truth is. No one does. It's a cosmic joke. A wise man once said: 'If someone wrote a book that was totally honest, it would be a masterpiece'. So this is what I am attempting. I'm not so sure it will be a masterpiece though. I want to tell you of the people in my life, and the stories I have invented. How different stories have interwoven into other stories, and how my mind is now a quagmire of varying sentiments and activity. Every mental vision within my brain is surely there for a reason? After a lengthy meditation of how thought operates once, I realised that a lot of it is based on association. But where does my series of associations lead me to be? What am I meant to do in this place? What can I do, in order to achieve? What do I want to achieve? Why do I feel trapped in a matrix of spectres, phantoms and people's judgements? Why do people rarely say what they are really thinking? What wrong did I do to justify this contamination of the brain? So I'm writing this letter / book to you as an attempt to compose an original piece of writing... One not confined to typical structure... The reason I have done this is to give you an insight into the way I look at the world, and I believe it is a form of writing that seeks to defy convention or narrative, and branch out into a more random stream of elements.

Last night, I was speaking to a man where I work. I don't know his name. I was explaining how life is mainly boring, or terror. From my point of view, this is something I've had to experience for ten years. The only rare escape from tedium and the flow of random thought imagery into an ecstatic state of mind is usually via the smoking of the ganja. I'm not allowed to smoke it anymore though. Mortals cannot understand its latent psychological effects. My parents think it's bad for me. Personally, it sends me into supersonic freeform cosmic hyperspace of hilarity, wonder, awe, and poetic mystery. I have often felt like a divine being when on the substance. I have golden soul pulses, and a circus of mental visions and insights. I get ideas that make me feel like a genius. It is my favourite escape. It's like heaven at times. No wonder Governments ban it... Just imagine a society where people were officially allowed to think like divine beings and live in a beautiful astral place of wondering freedom where music sounds like the messages of angels, and superpowers become the norm. No, no... We can't have society's populace living with expanded minds. They must be regulated, controlled, enslaved, so that those in charge reap the rewards and live their life of riches. (Empty riches more often than not... admittedly).

No, no... We can't have families jumping up and down giggling and feeling like they're in paradise, when the media constantly warns us of a whole host of dangers we must be alert to. 'Be vigilant!' 'Don't do this, don't do that'. 'Do this, do that'. Commands, rules, laws, thought control, brainwashing, indoctrination, conforming to the system... Prison.

I'm planning to escape... but I need what I deride in order to escape (perhaps you consider me a hypocrite?). I need the credits to freedom. The money. The dirty, filthy *moolah*. It's not an obsession. I certainly don't love money. In fact, I look down upon money. The credits. The freedom credits. Paper and metal tokens created by the state so that people might receive goods and services. I have to work for £5 an hour just to afford a packet of fags, and I am thirty, with a degree.

No... No more... I want plenty of freedom credits so I can get into a higher echelon of the prison. I don't want to be a low-grade prisoner anymore. I want to be a 'prison ideology generator'. I want to allow some to escape... but I need the credits. I need those pieces of paper with Beth's face on it to climb the rungs, and grant me power. Power is not freedom... but it is better than being stuck in a lower echelon cell (you might know it by its politically correct term: 'house') with only limited freedoms.

They call me schizophrenic because I had escaped the true way of legislated obedience long ago. I had boarded the alpha train to interstellar consciousness zone, and I had psychologically exploded. I'd been a big fish, in a small pond. Now I'm a small fish, in a big pond. It's not even a pond. It's more of an ocean. And I'm a tiddler. A tadpole. A useless little baby fish frantically swimming mentally in order just to find some understanding. We have a bar in the ocean prison... It's called a pub, but it's full of inmates who seem to lack any kind of higher understanding or vision. My parents, too... they're some of the most caged of all. My mother is interesting about 1 part in a 1,000. My father can be great, but he can also be nasty. And all the other inmates I meet are subjected to the jail of their own insecurity and mediocrity. It's hard to explode. No one wants to make a scene.

LOVE IN THE PRISON OF PSYCHOSIS

Celebration of anything is kept to a sober, quiet satisfaction. It's all very English. The media control system has ensured that we cannot unleash what we might be capable of. It's cranial Alcatraz for the civilised, and heaven for the wicked. Sure... it is an open prison... we can wonder into the commerce areas of the prison freely... but if you try to talk about something interesting to one of the prison staff, they look at you like you're a freak.

Mention 'the phenomenon of psychic astral interchange of two bonded freedom dreamers' to the lady at the local stationers, and she thinks you're barking mad. Poor woman. So trapped in her own prison and delusion that she knows what is real, that she doesn't even know the very basics of how to find freedom. True freedom. The freedom to feel divine and glowing with the almighty power of golden self-actualisation on an epic level. The place only heroes know... I knew it deeply once... But like Icarus, I flew too close to the sun, and landed crash, bang, wallop back into the psychotic prison. My parents had their cell upgraded, for sure... Our family cell costs about a million in freedom credits, but it's not the nirvana I sought. It's the physical embodiment of my father's slavery. It's the produce from most of his life wearing the prison slave costume for his particular department and busting a gut so that he can feed the family he created.

We have most things... all the material goodies that society creates to make the prison more complex and efficient, but I'm still caged... Caged in my body, my brain, and my cell... lusting to get high again, and enter the apotheosis of the legends. Where angels play euphonies no one else has heard, and you cannot stop laughing at the glory of the miracle of the universe. The zone where you actually feel you understand what God thinks. The zone where 'love and peace' seems to make so much spiritual sense as a political concept that you can't believe we don't have a bunch of hippies in Government.

Of course... They won't want to publish this... it's too 'far out'... They only publish stuff they deem as something that will maintain the mental prison structure. "All inmates must be focused, law abiding, disciplined, logical, and not unfurl their true souls, for fear of sectioning."

That seems to be the prison maxim. They're the confines by which the inmates are housed. Feed them fantasy... but don't let them do drugs. Let them smoke and drink and eat crap... but don't let them get high (because it's bad for their health). Don't let them smoke in bars and pubs because it's unhealthy (but build more roads and cars so that we can pollute the world even more).
Funny, isn't it? Asthma cases have gone up by 300% in the last ten years...and it ain't nothing to do with smoking in pubs. Cars are necessary though... The prison can't continue to operate peacefully unless the convicts are allowed to use the prison transportation system to get to their places of slavery, in order to work for the screws.

LOVE IN THE PRISON OF PSYCHOSIS

The screws aren't free either though, and they know it. There is limited freedom in this prison, except for the illusion of imaginative freedom the system propagates, and the freedom many enjoy should they break house rules, and smoke that blessed herb. Then... Even then... due to the oppression of rules and regulations, the great expanse of the mind can collapse into chronic paranoia and mental illness. This isn't the drug per se. The drug affects millions of people in positive ways. It's the psychology of that prisoner whilst influenced by the drug from his experience going through a personal series of mind considerations forged from his own understanding of living in the prison.

I know... because I've been there. The voices seek to celebrate or damn you. The phantoms of the unknown surround the spell that weaves your lack of understanding, and spins your neurons into new paths of synapse exploding confusion. Who is he? Who is she? What does he want? What does she want? What's he really thinking? What's she really thinking? Who does he work for? Who does she think she is? It's a complete anarchy of thought, and a complete concentration camp of actually exuded information. This dichotomy presents a dual world situation. The inner and the outer spaces. Where only the bravest of the brave (of which there are very few) venture out to expand our lives with missions of cultural relevance that augment the prisons walls with pretty posters, excellent books and the prison radio with happy songs. They then get taken to the Olympus area, where they are allowed to play live once in a while, to the prisoners, who dance and celebrate them, and think they're Gods... like the simpleminded Greeks and Romans, creating a new mythology.

Sure... the prison's artwork has given us the illusion that there is more freedom... but it's simply a regulating body endorsing the ability of some chosen inmates to express themselves for the sake of making sure not everyone goes mad. Half the people expressing themselves however, are the ones other people deem mad. Or is everyone mad? The human zoo... Neurosis, paranoia, insecurity, warped emotions, and dark, dark lust collide and construe in an epic struggle to maintain the prison status quo. What is the most normal thing in this day and age? I'll tell you the most normal thing... to have the discussion with someone that 'there is no normal'. This is so normal, that its paradox is elementary.

I met one of my favourite prisoners yesterday... His name is Mateus. He is a dude. He chose to eat a casserole with his new girlfriend at the local prison pub. It was good to see him again, although he's getting very stressed because he hardly has any freedom credits, even though he busts a gut. God dam it... When will we be set free? When will we be so wealthy that we will run the prison, and be able to decide who is allowed what, when and why? They seek to tell us we're too psychotic in

LOVE IN THE PRISON OF PSYCHOSIS

our division to be granted excess freedom passes. Lots of the time, most freedom credits go to the really sinister visionaries who know how to keep our prison a mighty influence for control in the world. Gunrunners, lawmakers, ideology enhancers, fantasy makers, screws, and electronics experts... They earn the big freedom credits. The psychotics get pittance. We're hardly allowed money to spend on alcohol, one of our few treats while we wait out our life sentence.

Only the best stock gets to live the great life. The life of fame and riches beyond that of the caged, where they have proved to be so powerful, strong and talented that they enhance the illusion so much that they are taken into the place of earthly wonders... Sure... it's still a part of the program, but they get the best of the coding... They get all the great stuff... Total immersion in all the fruits others have slaved for... Upgrades galore. Lauded as the prison saviours, they create a little eddy of optimism that there is a place to escape to for a small duration of time that captures the zeitgeist. Then, making sure the whole flurry of dreams is controlled technologically by the mind regulators. Once that eddy of hope has passed its little zenith of reverie, it is carefully moulded into another form of controlled thought using a series of exceptionally clever methods. E.g. 'antithesis genre phase cancellation enhancement' or they increase nefarious foreign data to suggest that other prisons are far starker than our own.

The lights light for a moment, then dwindle, and conform once they've got all the things they dreamt of. Only a handful of inmates manage this 'Life seize', and in this letter to you, I am hoping you might be able to help me get mine.

Sure... I'm digging a tunnel. I'm blowing a hole in the wall with literary TNT... But I've got to get out... I'm going madder than ever, and I'm not even on narcotics. My parents are so brainwashed, they won't even let me talk about what I want to talk about. They don't like new ideas... They don't understand them... They want commercialism ('Commercialism' is the euphemism for 'totally approved prison media for the masses'). It's almost always escapist because they want you to escape in your mind, so you're not concentrating on 'the reality' the whole time... But, after I spoke to one of my prison friends who helped in the science department, he explained how reality itself is now questioned by the highest figures in the land. The very fact that Queens, Princes, Bishops and Politicians are all questioning reality makes for one of two situations I can foresee:

1) They're going to make things even worse.
2) We might finally get a great escape.

But where to? The Internet has electronically housed most minds. Our information is all being stored in the massive computer labyrinth of data that will keep our futures pulsing on a server somewhere in Ohio. It's the foundations of the epic world siege. A whole series of nations could be wiped out in one day, when the main structure is finally in place. I have to get this message to you, my friend, because I need you on my renegade team. We need to understand what is really going on here. I can't tell you in concise English, because if the screws found out what I've stumbled upon, they'd take me out... Suffice to say, read the 'art of war'... Get a basic understanding of the power of networks, communications systems, and the power of information theory, and we have the beginnings of an apocalypse the likes of which will make World War II look like a fisty cuffs in a kindergarten playground.

Even if there was an escape... Where would we escape? We're one planet... In deep space. Most of it under strict authorised control now... I don't want to live on a polar icecap or in a desert for the rest of time. They've made sure that the ideological prison is now more luxurious than the totally untouched areas by man... but that's all part of the trick... It's all part of the scam... A cosy incubation system for the slaves. Keep them happy, keep them producing, but whatever you do... don't tell them the truth... because that'll send them mad... Allow them to travel abroad to feel free, and then watch as most of them transport little England to a sunny, foreign resort for a brief hiatus from the enslavement. Plug them into the entertainment network, and reflect their own earthly pleasures like a mirror of the psyche.

So, I take my work back underground, to stop it from falling into the wrong hands. I abide by the laws for a time, whilst secretly scheming through a method by which I can earn enough freedom credits to create my own illusion. I have a few allies, who appreciate my methods... but they're often on the perimeters of the prison society. Clever, sneaky, they venture into the ultra dimension whenever possible, and because they're strong, they know how to keep free from the screw's chastisements. I was unlucky. I did too much, too quickly. I spent a week on LSD once in order to find enlightenment. It worked, and I reached the apex of consciousness, but it came at a price. I felt the power of the most awesome divinity, and realised a millions insights in a split second. Do you know what that feels like? It is impossible to explain... I try to, but it all comes out in an abstruse garbled mess, where I can never know exactly what is real, what is not real, where to begin or where to stop.

I'm in a position where I don't even know if I'm totally sane or totally mad. What is sanity? What is 'reasonable thinking'? How can one weigh the currency of a thought? I see all the inmates wondering the corridors of the prison, and I wonder what they're really thinking. Perhaps they are all insane, and see sanity as insanity? How on earth can sanity be a concept if evolution is real? The very notion of evolution suggests to me that were we to be primal animals, then 'sanity' as a conception is a state sponsored conditioned myth used as a thought control mechanism in order to maintain social harmony. How can a biological computation system (the brain) know what sanity is when it is merely cultivated from cells for millennia? The idea that this natural aspect of life has some kind of reasoned coding sequence built into its processing capacity seems deeply illogical, unless you believe it's part of a grander design. Throughout history, people have presumed insanity, yet histories long trail of stories suggest to me there is no overriding hypothesis that can be deemed as 'sane'. Science, religion, literature, art, music, technology... it's all polarised, varied, morphing into new ways, like evolution itself. So where does a constant, which sanity must be, come in this expanse of time? Millions of people thought Hitler was a genius, let alone sane... But with hindsight, the world shudders at what that supposedly 'sane' man thought. On the other hand, many believed Christ was crazy. What does this tell you about people's understanding of sanity and insanity? THAT'S insane!

So now I'm at work in another cell. I'm doing my daily chores so that I might have shelter and eat. I am at a video shop... Or, as it is really called, a 'big brother audio visual morality coding bureau.' I sit alone, typing this letter so that we might find a purpose in our lives. Something to mean something. Something to tell, at least, one powerful message – however small. I smile at the other inhabitants of the town, but I don't know them from Adam. A guy from the meat-dispensing department waved to me today as I parked my road vessel, and I smiled back. I then thought about flicking him the finger, and then I thought 'why?' He's done nothing wrong to me, and he always seems friendly. I must be turning into a bastard. The idea just popped in there. I haven't had a kiss from a girl in over two months, and I'm beginning to think my house is bugged by MI5. The voices are taunting me, telling me that they want to see me beaten up, raped, and murdered... because I know too much. They are sickening minds, with inherent demonic properties utilising their despotic grasp on my reason to force me to conform to their iniquitous methods. So... I acquiesce covertly to their subjugation for a while... but I have a gift that many don't proffer... I can think outside the norm, and write.

I suppose my own psychohistory tells another story... I was raised in an elitist establishment. By all rights, I should be rich by now thanks to a decent education. But I found the world too much of a cosmic mystery to operate successfully once I had ingested so many psychoactive materials. I'm almost a down and out. I hardly ever wash my hair or brush my teeth. I bath... sure... for over an hour a day, for it is where I commune with the divinity in a sober fashion in deep meditation, but the rest of the day is a series of bombarding senses receiving data upon data of vast information, the likes of which I could never process into one defined state of intelligent reason. Hence the way I'm writing this letter... So that you might know how the mind truly flows. It is not bound by the convention of literature, where a model for an elaborate agenda is enforced in order to convey a particular story in order to explain succinctly a fiction. This is not fiction... This is a mind trying to tell the truth... This is an inhabitant of the southern realms seeking to make known his comprehension in a fabricated society of confusion and bewilderment. When the ladies and gentlemen you see in town look at you, what are they thinking? Do they want you dead? Do they like you? What is there to like in me? I am a psychotic who only just managed to escape sectioning during the crisis years when the world teetered on the brink of collapse.

The anarchists loved that of course... They relished the idea of the prison totally collapsing, and world being thrown into chaos. I enjoy neither... I desire a middle path... complexity. But, you have to give credit where credit is due... The system maintains dominion and order. Sure... it's full of evil swine, but there's also some merit in a jail that continues to oppress itself so efficiently in the name of survival. Like a massive multifaceted organism, it oozes through time forever stamping on the threats and consuming and consuming for no other apparent reason than to propagate and consume more. I am opposed to total anarchy as well as I am opposed to tedium. Anarchy would be the polar opposite, and yet even worse potentially... It is a non-workable idea, which would herald only a few enthusiasts.

So where do I go? Which ideology do I subscribe to? Who is right, and who is wrong? Who is really intelligent, and who is not? Questions, questions, questions... The music continues to play, and I consider the artist's state of mind. What is his *raison d'etre*? Why does he speak to a million people and others speak to none? Can the future of politics be galvanised by the bass line of a rock track, or the riff of a synthesiser tune? Music shapes the prison agenda in so many ways... but what is its essential synthesis? Confusion... it seems... Part of the grand plan... Pump the prisoners' minds with sensual stimulation, and they will continue to emanate good feelings / positive vibes. This then enhances the illusion that we're free, but according to St. John the Divine: we're only ever heading towards the apocalypse... One man's freedom is another man's Satanism. One man's dictatorship is another man's paradise. Causality, duality, the impossibility of equality. It all stacks up to become a monolith of wonder and mystification. The wisest have engineered this on purpose I believe... to keep us hungry, wanting, producing, even ready to die in the name of abstract notions. The absurdity! When will we find a singularity of deep truth? What is the aforementioned organism's real purpose? I suspect something terrible... A maze of thought processes all rippling around their cells with no particular rhyme or reason to the whole thing...

LOVE IN THE PRISON OF PSYCHOSIS

Yet, with this mass of media enforced information and illusion, I still feel caged... It's because I understand the trick... The grand design... and that makes me dangerous if I'm not committed to the allegiance... So I step outside the circuit of the power wielders, and pen this missive... WE MUST TRY TO KNOW WHAT WE ARE NOW... Many don't... Inmates resort to drink, drugs, sex, escapism, fetishes, violence, vanity, fiction, self-harm, perversion... Many of us cannot take the pressures of the modern world... so the tensions build like a bubble subliminally, and it is only thanks to the goodness in faith that we haven't all collapsed into a swamp of physical insanity long ago.

Thus, we cage ourselves in order to survive. But is a caged soul worth surviving? What is its point, if it is not helping to build and improve the prison? A fat, consuming, nobody who simply takes up resources and doesn't offer any kind of talent seems to be anathema to value. We let them consume and become grotesque, and they then call themselves America – Land of the free. Free? What is freedom without dope? It is inferior... The ganja is the true liberation of the mind and spirit, and a theory goes that Jesus was enlightened thanks to his use of it. It is considered by some that it is one of the ingredients of the holy anointing oil described in the book of Exodus. In English, it is translated as 'fragrant cane', (from the Hebrew Keenah Bosem) but some have considered this to be cannabis... This would explain a hell of a lot, let me tell you. Not to the cowardly religious fanatics who are largely a Christian through no other reason than ignorance and stygiophobia, but to those spirits whose souls have become supreme under the influence, and know the states of utopian genius it can manifest in the right people.

Sure… for some, it has negative effects, but again, this says something about the person, not necessarily the drug. But no… The system wants you plugged in, zoned out, and obedient to moneymaking. Money won't save you… So what does one do? We're locked into a dependency. A dependency on the system to make sure we're going to be okay, so we capitulate to tedium and sit back. Most people talk tedious crap. They don't have the nerve, the imagination or the wit to discuss things at a higher level. They simply discuss the mundane… adding to the sense of a prison. Housed, self imposed avatars of the universe all talking platitudes and clichés. The inhabitants… All infected by system indoctrination - robots of a form. So I dwell in the shadows, watching, listening – planning.

The way I am writing this is not the methods of a madman… It is a different concept in writing. If we cannot escape the system, because we ARE the system, and we depend on the system to support who we are, we can, at least, open channels of higher discourse. An enlightening conversation in a jail is still a good conversation. I pray that I won't be relegated to maximum security if this missive

LOVE IN THE PRISON OF PSYCHOSIS

falls into the wrong hands... But I have to express myself... I have to explain my mind, so that others might understand me clearly, and then know how to treat me. But will you know how to treat me? Or will you loathe my every utterance on this page...

This is: "X" – the abstract value.

X, in this instance, equals 'this point in time'.

'This point in time' will be different for you when you read it... For every person who reads it, their 'X' will be a unique situation. Different minds, different stories, different tastes, different ideas, different status... a different 'X'. So, your exegesis of this experimental narrative is thus 'your X', and that is something I cannot possibly know what it is like to experience. Therefore, this is a one-route path from me, branching out to you, creating, hopefully, a series of Xs. Only if this missive becomes successful, will each 'X' for each different prisoner be valued at something, and then grow to be a network of hypothesis and personal belief like a massive relay of connectivity of concept, as long as you remember your 'X'. What will be the first opinion you have after your 'X'? Will you share it with someone else? A tirade of X points could create a pattern... a new pattern... a random sequencing of moments carved from this very trigger point. Your 'X' is determined by your own conditioning; however, I don't wish to sully your 'independent' thought by using suggestion. So I will not continue to speak on the matter of the 'X'... It is a special thought you should write down here, and keep for further analysis in the future:

So now we return to the moment... the Post–X situation, where X is a possibly totally unique value. I have begun to set free your mind... Now compute the following equation:

$X > Y$

Where 'Y' is the next thought you have. Association? Is it associated? Write down Y:

We now have X and Y... and two different thoughts. How much of it is affected by the words on this page? How much of it is associative? How varied or surreal is the disparity between X and Y? Now... what is the currency of those two factors? What do they say to you, as an individual? How bound by my terms are your thoughts? No doubt, you might be thinking of Y prominently as a mathematical symbol, and are perhaps verging towards maths as a consideration, given that we're now dealing with algebraic notions. But this is only a 'maybe'.

STOP.

Aphid kneecap gel.

There... I've implanted a surreal image into your mind to change your thought process. See? Now I have complete control of your mind. This is how media mind control works at a basic level. You came to this book seeking answers. I have given you no answers. I have just controlled your mind for a moment. Thus, I am creating your thought process as I write these words... but you have chosen to be inculcated up to this point with my conditioning. Are you in my mind, or am I in your mind? This is how it all works, and why the Bible and Koran are both ancient programs. I am zooming left, right, up and down in my thinking to take you on a ride... A mental excursion into a new way of thought... But will the system like my thought process? The test of the freedom of the prison will dictate the level by which I am conditioning you. However, who on earth says I don't have the right to condition you? And who the hell, if not me, DOES have the right to condition you?

Break the stream... close your eyes, and think of something YOU desire...

Got it? Got that thing in your mind you desire?

See... I'm still conditioning you... but this time, by proxy. YOU have just thought of the one thing you desire because I instructed you to do so, using a separate variable. Thus, was it a personal thought based on freethinking? No... I instructed you to imagine whatever it is in your own life that you desire so much, a core and much-mused on dream... So, if I can take you so easily to that warm mental hemisphere where you recline in the notions of dreamlike 'if onlys'... Where else can I take you?

Hawaii?

Now I see the imagery in your head... Most of it will be clichéd... Most of it will be typical ideas of dancing girls with flowers, palm trees, surf, beaches, seafood, sun, islands, volcanoes, and the 49th state of America. (There will be political residue attached to this trigger due to system inculcation). If you've been before, there might be a less state enforced symbolism for you... A personal memory, perhaps.

However, let us step outside of that cliché... Keep your 'idea' of Hawaii, and now place in your mind's eye a German on a pogo stick singing 'Tie me kangaroo down boy' with a turnip attached to his head.

Alakazam...

Original thought implant generated to all people who read this... Why? Why not? A form of freedom, yet for none of you is this really freedom. Now, you all have a similar idea in mind, one that I have designed. That's what I do, design ideas... And I bet, due to the weight of what you have been reading and the focus by which you should be reading this section, all of you who have got this far will never think of Hawaii in the same way

LOVE IN THE PRISON OF PSYCHOSIS

again because of the concentrated effect I have implanted in you.

Aren't you glad it was surreal and harmless?

It could be far worse. I could implement something terrible... Something absolutely horrific, that you would reel in fear and throw this missive away. Thus, 'harmless and surreal' generates something pleasing in this instance. Something almost amusing that will have you at ease, but I have already planted that seed of doubt... That seed within this paragraph that something terrible might lie behind the next page. A concept so utterly vile, so utterly shocking, that your mind, while being controlled by me, will be uncontrollably taken to a place you never wanted to go. Sure... you can stop reading, but I've got many of you hooked now, haven't I? You might even be looking forward to that terrible thing... or you might be biting your lip, wondering if you should read on... Now I've caused a disparity in psychology: the difference between mental agendas. Some will want to know, some won't want to know... Explorers and hiders. Will you continue to venture with me? Are you brave, or are you worried? Are you excited, or do you think I am insane?

Come... this way... watch the marbled flooring, it costs quite a bit.

There... now we're in my mind mansion, and I can show you yet more aspects of your own existence that combined with mine, are creating a psychological bridge of philosophical discovery. Do you like me controlling your thoughts like this? Or do you find it irritating? Am I annoying you?

Here... think of a rose... In a garden of sunshine...

I hope I have furnished your imagination now with something more pleasing to the soul. It's nice in the garden, isn't it?

BUT IT'S STILL A CLICHÉ...

I am going to place a green swan sitting on a nest of rock and roll fliers in that garden, right next to the mental image of you with the rose. Now what do you think? How is the association? It's certainly a different idea to the cliché I had caused you to stumble on. Name the swan... Give it a moniker.

Write that name down here:

Now I have just asked you to consider a new thought. This is not necessarily an associative value. It will be very much an independent, personal name that might mean something to you. There will be a small amount of associative properties due to the nature of it being a bird and the potent idea of 'rock and roll' and 'flowers', but the name you create is very much a thought designed on your own terms. BUT, I bet you it's a name you've used before, or really like. I might be wrong, but I imagine you've given it a name that either:

a) Means something to you at a level you don't even necessarily understand.
b) Describes quasi-phonetically your symbolic interpretation of that image.

Either way... this is a thought process that although I have triggered, YOU have designed via my instruction. However, the name is likely to be known to you, unless it is a surreal nonsensical word. And thus, ignoring the latter point, if it *is* known to you, then why do you think this name which you've learned through your travels through life has such deep meaning in your ideas? Why do you appreciate this name?

I am now wondering what varied streams of names might be used as you all choose different names in different parts of the prison, in different mental imagery.

I am growing tired of this little exercise, so I'm going to quantum leap.

"Writing for the 21st Century"

Where now? Where on earth can we go? Let me tell you the things that have spiralled through my mind in the last minute:

Sugababes – push the button

Anatomy of a whale.
Calendar of motorcycle events.
Dukes of hazard.
Playschool dumplings.
All out frenzied waltzing.
Serene pullovers.
Tarmac genius.
Quality processing.
Essential sounds of the Victorian period.
Rubbish tips.
Varying shades of the colour blue.

What is all that about? This is the vague wanderings of a mind that hasn't got stoned in a while. It was so much fun, let us do it again. I'll just sit here, tuned into my brain, and write down all the things that come to mind in the next minute:

Ready? Go...

Pushover bullies.
Random harpsichords.
Winnie the Pooh in trouble.
Secondary equations.
Foolish Mexican.
Damn the current.
Flaying soldiers of ineptitude.
Difficult crossroads.

Eh??? These are the mysterious elements that comprise two minutes of my thinking on a random day in October. You probably think I'm talking complete crap, but isn't the rest of the writing so far structured fairly logically?

If you think 'yes', then I would suggest that, even though I was attempting to write the truth earlier, the last series of lines is closer to the truth than any of the premeditated and purposefully designed writing that precedes it. So what we are left with are at least the following potential situations:

1) I am simply writing selfishly with an agenda, in order to control your minds in a certain way; masquerading as someone who deludes himself or herself into thinking they know the truth.
2) The truth is actually far more surreal and bizarre than most people are prepared to admit. ('Truth' in this instance is 'thought').
3) The 'truth' is an unfathomable term, something that even in 2,000 years, *anno domini*, we cannot begin to comprehend due to the sheer complexity of the universe and all its components.
4) This is my truth… tell me yours…

Even with such free flowing mental activity, it has been 30 years in the making, so what does that tell me about my current situation – and what do you think of my current situation? Am I lying to you? No…

This is the free stream of my own personal thought process, and yet, much of those previously mentioned random thoughts are possibly pseudo-nonsensical. However, during those two one minute exercises, I conjured a number of images in your mind – very few of which were clichés. It was all triggered by something though... but triggered by what? I simply sat in the video department with these words swelling up in my cranium at a seemingly random level. What on earth are they supposed to mean? I don't know... I can make a supposition, but I cannot know for sure.

However, it is going to take a giant leap of the imagination to know what to do with a mind that works this way. Perhaps we all work that way, subconsciously, but we are not prepared to admit it. Or, perhaps, I have entered a deeper sphere of my mind due to my experiences, psychohistory and nurturing? Maybe this is how we should write from now on... No longer presuming that basic logic is the correct thought process, but that a free formed mind in chaos is closer to the zenith of consciousness when applied to an earthly atmosphere of an infinite number of atoms all operating together in the cohesion of mammoth interconnectivity. To extrapolate from the fundamentals of 'logic' (which in itself only tends to the knowledge of other logical minds, and a basic understanding of earth's behaviour through experience), and insist that everything noted down should follow a form by which we can muster true reason seems to be the bricks that build the prison walls. When one knows, as I do, that there *are* phenomena in spiritual existence, then this immediately throws the concept of logic into question. How then, do we find out the truth of the phenomena I have encountered? (Such as visions, O.B.Es, enlightenment). How can we step into that higher dimension, where the notions of divinity hail from, and learn of those mental truths that have caused me to spiral out of the mundane and into a reality, dripping in revelation? Does 'genius tarmac', or 'damn the current' contain deeper messages that should be heeded? Is it my conditioning in the prison all these years that have caused my thoughts to operate so surreally, or am I really closer to the notion of 'perfect consciousness' than others might be?

To me, this is a higher form of freedom... but a solitary one – for now. Also, as it is so potentially nonsensical at this juncture... what is its point? What if everyone spoke like this? What kind of conversation would people have? I know a woman who got a first at an art degree, and the work she produced was complete crap... but then... isn't it the foundation of the kind of thinking that this book is seeking to espouse?

Let us trickle on down stream to a little tuft of grass, where we can have a moment to reflect on what this is all about. What is it to you? Is it gibberish? Or a happy and unique crusade into the mind of a different spirit? I hope I'm not being heretical in anything I might be saying... but then, there is no greater brainwasher than that of religion.

Let us look at some of the absurdities of religion:

1. The concept of hell juxtaposed with that of a loving God.

This whole idea is so utterly appalling to me, that I cannot fathom it. How on earth can a God of love subject millions of souls (as it says in the bible) to eternal damnation in hell fire? What monstrous notion of barbaric punishment is this? I laughed my head off once while having a theological debate with a Christian. I mentioned my disgust at this concept, and she replied: "Does not a parent punish their child when they have transgressed?" To which I replied: "Not by throwing them on a bonfire for eternity!"

What a complete joke. There are thousands of religious people around the world (and ones choice of religion is often largely based on a matter of geography rather than intellectual understanding or theological reasoning). Some Christians believe all non-Christians are going to hell. Muslims, Hindus, Jews, Buddhists... no matter what alien religion, devised completely from no actual concrete evidence, all burn in eternity, for reasons such as not having even heard of Jesus Christ. This is the most absurd thing I have ever come across. It's worse than Nazism. A 'loving Christian' will, depending on their philosophy, seek what is essentially a mammoth genocide, simply because the person they are seeking to send to hell for eternity thinks differently. And what is their defence? One of the lines is "Through the blood of Christ, we are saved," or "I am saved because I am cleansed in the blood of the lamb".

What the dickens is that supposed to mean? Don't give me any weird arguments... I won't have it... It is totally weird and nonsensical hocus-pocus. How can a man, divine or not, save people by being tortured and killed? I know some arguments for this, like 'It was so God could experience the suffering of man'. "He died so that we might be saved" – saved from what? An evil concept engineered by a God (who no one has seen) of love? What on earth is this rubbish all about? Hell? Justice? I wouldn't even send Hitler to hell. I might imprison him in a maximum-security utility for years and years and years, but hell? The idea is as bad as anything Satan might try to do. Can you imagine anything more evil than burning someone alive for all time? That's the kind of stuff serial killers think about. Is God the ultimate serial killer? Have people, who were born much earlier, been burning all these years, simply because they were born into another time? Please... What a joke.

2. You must be circumcised to enter the kingdom.

Eh??? Although this is largely more a Judaic custom than Christian (as St. Paul changed that aspect of the scriptures), what on earth is that meant to mean? You cannot find the favour of God, unless the prepuce, which you are naturally born with, is removed when born? What?!? How on earth can you take the Bible seriously when it says this? It's like saying: "You're born with four fingers and a thumb, but the thumb must be removed if you wish to find salvation in the name of a metaphysical idea". I must stifle the laughing now, for this is so absurd that I can no longer contain my joy at the possibility of there being nothing out there at all, if it's so damn strange. Don't give me arguments about hygiene either, because if God did make us – as some people believe – why on earth give us a foreskin if it is to be removed the moment we're born?

3. Noah's ark.

There is a church in Brighton that is built to the same specifications of the ark. (Using the measurements gleaned from Genesis). I have visited it. No way on 'Gods' good earth could a building of that size, large as it is, house two of every animal. Also… in all these years of religious debate and global argument over a 'big idea', no one I have ever met has pointed out one obvious fact. Aside from the idea that Noah must have visited Australia long before Captain Cook, in order to save kangaroos, koalas, duck billed platypuses and co, no one has seemingly bothered to think: 'but what about insects'? There are over 5,000 different species of beetle alone. Are you seriously suggesting that Noah collected in excess of two of every kind of the millions of different species of insect, including the varieties we haven't even discovered yet? You have got to be kidding. One Christian, whose L.E.D. wasn't the brightest bulb on the dash, said 'God helped Noah'. Oh right! Well… that's handy. God saves one family, and millions of different kind of insects (which would have had to be housed all individually in protective containers, so as to not be eaten by all the other insect eating / carnivorous animals on the ark), but slaughters the rest of the world, killing far more than Hitler ever did? Thank you God of love!

By the way, Lord, can you tell me why you're so inconsistent? To start with, you're an angry, jealous, punishing God, and then, thanks to Jesus, you become all loving. How do you think people who were living before your personality change felt? Does placing one's penis into the vagina of a woman who is not officially married to the man *really* require such brutal chastisement as hell fire, when you yourself are guilty of genocide, murder, all manner of confusion, wars seemingly without end, famine, pestilence, hypocrisy and plagues?

4. The concept of love.

The Christian concept of love is a right hoot. They are inculcated by freaks that believe in a book full of holes, and from then on have changed their attitude to people. If you're gay, you go to hell (in some of their minds). Even, according to the English translation (and some people will argue there are problems with translations, but frankly, if God is so supreme and all knowing, surely he would have known his book was going to be translated into the second most widely spoken language on the planet?) if you're effeminate, not even gay... you go to hell. This is why I liken God to Hitler, for he did stuff like that. Buddhists are not off the hook either. Some of them will ignore and deride a handicapped person because 'he was bad in a previous life'. What? Hasn't the poor person got enough to worry about, without being told by some high-minded weirdo that he shouldn't be helped, because of something he did 'in a previous life'? Where is the evidence for this ever taking place? I don't think that would go down too well in court.

("Why did you ignore this cripple when he was dying?"

"Because he was a murderer in a previous incarnation two hundred years ago in Beijing, m'Lord.").

He's been judged as an 'evil person' simply for being born a cripple to some Buddhists. Poor chap... as if life wasn't hard enough, some deluded freak inspired by an Eastern idea, which is just as potentially ludicrous as any other, dismisses him as evil – no doubt walking off thinking to himself, 'I'm healthy, I'm good, Buddha will be pleased that I've ignored that paraplegic trying to move ten yards'.

LOVE IN THE PRISON OF PSYCHOSIS

As for Christian compassion, well... Some of them will love you if you say Jesus is your saviour (by some unfathomable means of being crucified, which funnily enough is one punishment you *could* survive, taking into account the nature of the penalty. I'd like to see him wake from the dead after a beheading), but if you question *their* interpretation of Jesus, even if you believe in Jesus in your own way, they'll be quite happy to sit back and imagine you burning for eternity in hellfire. Yeah, really nice people...

And what about Catholics and Protestants killing and hating each other? I don't think I've yet met a Christian who's managed to love their enemy. Let alone hating and loathing people on what is to all intents and purposes 'the same side' but with a few different policies and tribal totems. It seems that the basic mindsets of many imbeciles in society, who cling to religious concepts and yet fuel hatred, are the bi-product of poor education. "Think as I think, or be damned", they all seem to cry in polarised unison. What an elaborate tapestry of delusion! Only the seemingly wise, who are granted positions of authority within the prison ranking matrix, understand this most basic of fundamental hypocrisies. Yet, who is doing anything about it? Thankfully, the prison radio transmission system has agreed to promote, in general, an agenda that celebrates the ideology of 'love'. (All the music is generally fairly positive, in order to keep the inmates upbeat and efficient), but it is in the detail that both God and the Devil have been accused of operating (another strange contradiction). Listen to Radio 1 late at night and you will get an idea of what is really out there...lying in the cracks of the crazy mental paving. The demons, the mentally tortured, the vile, the wicked, the nefarious, the hateful... It should be called 'Satan FM' late at night. I imagine it's the elevator music to Hades, would such a horrendous concept ever be reality?

5. Muslim extremism

I watched the decapitation of Ed Berg on the Internet, and quite frankly, it was the most evil thing I've ever seen in my life. All in the name of a God, which recognises Jesus as a prophet, but of course, has different views on various matters. What a load of rubbish... As for flying planes into the twin towers, and killing thousands of people, since when did a 'religion' say it was right to kill people? It's one of the most nefarious crimes throughout time (although, of course, God and Moses get away with it – because they run the racket). Not only that, but when people complained about the behaviour of the Taliban, I was simply reminded of the Pentateuch. If the Jewish people today followed the laws of the Torah as strictly as they are written down in Leviticus and co., they'd be just like the Taliban. Death to gays, adulterers, blasphemers, etc.
Hold on a minute though... they can't eat pork... because God says so. But wait! Christians can eat whatever they like because God says so. But wait! Hindus can't eat beef, because cows are sacred.

LOVE IN THE PRISON OF PSYCHOSIS

And Muslims can't eat pork either… because God says so! But he said others could!
And after all this… which day is the real Sabbath? Friday, Saturday or Sunday? They can't all be right. Someone somewhere is going to be proved wrong one day and, considering the number of people involved in each religion that proselytises these concepts, that's a lot of people in the wrong…
(As an amusing aside, I met a Muslim once who said 'the world will end on a Friday'. To which I responded 'How do you know?' "Because it's the Sabbath", he replied).

6. The Garden of Eden.

Well… wasn't it nice for God to create a paradise for Adam and Eve. They were meant to live forever, until Eve bit the fruit from the tree of knowledge. (Talking snakes existed in Eden). Well… aside from blaming the fall of all men on a woman (which seems fairly misogynistic, to say the least), I have to say I'm rather pleased… or, according to the theory, I wouldn't have been born. So… thanks to Eve transgressing on a monumental level, (typical female minx, getting it on with the devil – saucy bint) billions of people have been born, which is cool because we now have a modern world full of great stuff. But the logic behind the argument that an entire massive planet was originally designed to house only two people in paradise – a paradise, might I add, that didn't even involve Haagen daz cookies and cream, the Internet, pizza, or the 'star wars saga' seems a trifle strange. Also, where did all the other people come from in Genesis? Did God make a load more people from the off-cuts? Where did they pop up from? Was Eve pumping them out in secret?

Some geneticists and anthropologists even claim that all people on the planet's DNA can be traced back to a man and a woman who walked out of Africa. Oh really? Everyone in the world's DNA has been tested, has it? And while I'm on the subject of evolution, exactly why is everything so precise in nature if evolution is as random and accidental as they suggest? A horse is a horse, a pig is a pig, an adder is an adder, a butterfly is a butterfly, a scorpion is a scorpion, etc. Surely, if evolution was true to form, they'd be a billion different amalgamations of varying species. Why are Gorilla's still around, if we evolved from them? Why don't we have a talking chimp? Where are the crossovers? I'm not convinced... The whole notion that we should believe either a) God made us (and according to the Koran, he made man in at least four different ways) or b) we evolved from monkeys. Both seem incredulous to me... Yet, one man reads a book that is well written and its arguments either logical or illogical, and suddenly, it's 'I know the truth!' and everyone gets in a heated debate, and sometimes fall out. Pricks. No wonder the prison has rarely large parties. Most people can't stand to listen to one another's religious views. Although I wouldn't go as far as Satre, and claim 'Hell is other people', I certainly think the bespectacled little bore had it too easy if he thinks that. My god... how easy was his life, if he thinks the idea of hell (a concept I have experienced for 8 hours on a far higher level of suffering) is simply someone in his local vicinity? He must have seen mankind as demons... Perhaps there is some truth to that, but they seem generally nice on the surface in the main. Perhaps Satre was just so socially inadequate that he brought out the worst in people. I happen to love many people and enjoy their company. It's hardly the evil conflagration of eternal flames that the term vicariously generates.

7. The Apocalypse

Well... you thought World War 2 was bad. You wait until you work out some of what the book of Revelation is on about. In one paragraph, it talks of wiping out a third of the world's population. Just like that. If that happened tomorrow, that would be two billion people. Two billion?? Furthermore, it mentions the rise of the anti-Christ, who is Satan... and he will mark the forehead or the right hand of everyone so that they may buy or sell'. Well... There are plenty of conspiracies on the Internet as to what this might actually mean, and considering we should really be on the look out for this kind of thing happening, it seems a bit of a bummer that the whole book is so ambiguous. I mean... The 'whole world', aside from a few Christians (who will be beheaded instead), will follow this 'man'? "And the number of the beast is

666". What on earth is that supposed to mean? Many theologians say that 7 is 'a holy number', and '6' is a sign of imperfection. How can a number, which is essentially a symbol that represents an amount, have moral properties?? Eh?? It's like saying: "the number 9 is very envious", or "The number 14 is racist". The more I study religion, and politics, the more I see how utterly absurd the world in which we live in is... and hence the reason they've created the prison...

With information like that flying about as though it is the word of a supreme being, no wonder everyone hates to talk about religion and politics, and instead gets high on drink and drugs and talks of breast enlargements, celebrities (the pantheon of the modern euhemerism), and where they went on holiday.

But it's not just believers who create a mishmash of anomalies and absurdities. Has millions of pounds really been invested into the mobile phone market so that my parents can send me a text from Majorca saying 'We're in a restaurant, and Ma is having an omelette, and I'm having the steak'. So what? Do I really need to know this information? Big fat hairy deal. Someone give me a joint, so I can commune with the universe at the level of a deity. THAT'S something to write home about... But no... I'm not allowed to enter the higher realms of the cosmic splendour... Logic, mendacity, insecurity, self-containment, tedium, and fake satisfaction must be a constant. My parents can't have their son actually finding something miraculous about life. It would be

LOVE IN THE PRISON OF PSYCHOSIS

awfully un-middle class. Let us make every day a mundane routine instead... Robots, conforming to a system of less than interesting agendas and precepts, whereby conversation in any form is guarded by the realities that one must not express higher beliefs for fear of being deemed 'invalid' ideologically by the screws.

Anyway... I rant, and I rant, and I rant... and the borders of my writing are still confounded by temporal limitations of my cognitive ability, for I am on medication to keep me sedated. (Not too high, not too low... but juuuuust mediocrity).

There is a rose between these thorns though... There is a diamond in this coalface of routine. There is a female dream whose beauty is so mesmerising, that she allows me to escape from the cells for a moment, and the 'do this, do that' command centre. She is one of the prison inmates of my sector. Although I am not allowed to go out with her, due to her decision that I am an inferior specimen who wallows in a mire of self-induced anguish. Every time I gaze upon her countenance, and see those solar eyes and beaming smile, I am taken for a second to Olympus. That place where the great escapes. Only vicariously, of course... but it is enough to keep up one's hope while waiting to die of boredom and old age in the prison.

I wrote her this letter… But I cannot give it to her. She would consider me more insane than all the other nutters:

Forest Zone,
Cell 37,
Sector SPX 2BH

The Setup

The spirits in the wind had informed Prince Nicholas that Princess Danni (whose regal authority had been granted unto her by him) had wanted him damned. Such soul wrecking data caused an onslaught of rage to filter about Prince Nicholas's shattered reality as he strove to maintain some semblance of meaning in a community that understood him not.

The passing of time, and the random and seemingly haphazard moments in one's personal existence collided to such an extent at this juncture that the Prince was forced to act. He knew Danni was young. Tender minds, in their folly, could not muster the ken that one so requires at any year, when met with a manifest onslaught of existences very nature. Therefore, Prince Nicholas of the south was moved to react to such a dastardly notion by which the lady he so adored should conclude to be a necessary cause, when he had done nothing but warrant her favour. He giggled at the experiences he had found on solo outings into the local community, and considered how those memories were housed in his cranium. He knew that a wealth of information had bypassed his retinas in the last half decade, but few moments were gilded and as cherished as those precious aspects of affection that he had solemnly enjoyed, as he quietly sat in the Judaic outpost of intoxication studying the luscious angel before his eyes.

He mused on the virtues of a young Cinderella whose pride was such that she dare not seek to grant his forward methods as valid, for he was a curious breed, and notorious for a plenitude of reasons (most originating from the amusing certitude that people could not comprehend his methods).

Prince Nicholas was so moved by such a genius incarnation of the local populace that he would wreck souls, destroy plantations, and damn hell it cause untold suffering was his beckoning of a kiss from such a wondrous female not be met with mutual regard. He had suffered the hypocrisy of the prisoners for so long, and faced the constant barrage of hatred for so many oscillations of molecules that he was forced to 'carpe diem', and react to this gross injustice with the grandeur of a saint possessed.

He had seen the young damsel... the princess she was (of the lower orders, but wielding enough charm, grace and professionalism to be granted due respect by the higher echelons) in her verdant chariot. Sure... many thought it silly to grant such terms to common ideas of what was what, but Prince Nicholas contained a sensory that was enhanced by the most virulent strain of potent knowledge. As he sat in his high chamber, his mind reeling with the latest in a pantheon of instruction from all manner of mortal men, he knew it was time to act... and, so doing, he conjured a plan that might indeed win the hand of the fair Danni.

She was shrewd though... She wasn't a slapper whose controversial parts dilated and pulsed for the very thumping of a solid member against those areas not discussed in polite society, with nothing to augment that pleasure but the barbaric code of the perverted infidel... (You might think me crude here... but am I fooled? No... I see the obsession with sex filter through society on a daily basis). She was a lady of class, whose original congenital fortunes of stature were admittedly humble, but she wielded so many gifts that Nicholas could not help but alight his being in her proximity. He had even met her parents, and enjoyed their spirit dearly... Enjoying both the humour of the paterfamilias, and the pure beauty of 'she who had housed that sacred zygote'.

Yes, yes... Nicholas wrote prose that few could react to when facing a multidimensional world of varying methods of communication, but Nicholas possessed gifts too, and, although he had squandered them in his naïve youth, he'd learned to harness the most basic of miracles with time. (Time being that treasured constant that all life was granted to experience somewhere in the annals of chronology, for a purpose as yet unknown by seemingly all of its inhabitants).

They came to the tavern of Moses in their droves at times… from all aspects of society's bizarre and wayward course. The kids would call him drunk, the wise would call him dangerous, the cowardly would call him arrogant, and the loving were his believers. But dear, dear Danni… Princess Danni (such a wondrous concept) could not dare imagine the potentiality of taking this one mystic's hand in love, and manifesting a union. She expected more from a suitor, and who could blame her? She was in charge of all the boons that a young dame might dream for, and, as such, could expect to court even the most fine and affluent natives of this green and pleasant province.

What would occur? What manner of chaos could endure, should these two disparate spirits be entwined? He knew she had rejected Principle Stuart for the pounding reveries of the nefarious infidel, in order to feel the contemporary, strident palpitations of a young jock consumed with vanity… But Prince Nicholas had seen through the heathen on that day that Danni remembered, and thus contaminated her reality with a certain blemish of discord that ricocheted through her very fibre, were her current beau not to be the Romeo of muscles and stock she had originally fantasised.

Sure... Nicholas was a wild man... a loose canon, a wild and crazed enlightened spirit pin-balling his way through the labyrinth of humanoids all spewing emotional filth in their desperate attempts to be granted authority by some individual they placed on a pedestal. But Prince Nicholas, as potentially mad as he was (and he knew he wasn't), merely chortled in his secret golden glow of divine manifestation as he watched their pathetic struggle to comprehend his cognitive explosions.

He had allies, as well as enemies. It was all working out to be yet another sad dimension in generations, whereby the wealth of lacklustre instruction of all souls had forged themselves to a point in the grand expanse of current purpose, that he acknowledged correctly that everyone was more or less 'full of shit'. The Asiatic units propagated their liquid, ebony gold, but still... What manner of meaning did this conjure for the occidental spawn that laughed and fornicated in their stupor as their delusion of this ephemeral matrix spun on a transient political fulcrum?

They continued in their hubris to indulge in the pleasures of sickening fantasies. The obsession with carnal activities beamed down upon their nefarious skulls as the prime source of cerebral

LOVE IN THE PRISON OF PSYCHOSIS

processing, but Prince Nicholas knew that this was a diabolical nonsense that would suffer its recompense in a posthumous dimension.

Make note... Prince Nicholas did not scribe these terms in order to vex or confuse the wonder of the Princess, but did so in order to promote an idea of what was 'virtuous England'. By generating a superhuman approach to biological form that had sadly been overlooked by the mass of irreligious non-entities that plagued this unique land, his apotheosis would take shape like a series of flanks upon a diamonds countenance. Each plateau of the multi-faced treasure was like a prism, thus symbolically representing a holistic mind of the dancing spectrum. If colour can be seen in the mind, then where is the light in the mind that provides this pigmentation? Is it via the eyes the mind learns the variance of hues? How does a brain, housed completely in a dark skull, render such tinctures from a mental process?

I digress...

Sure... in their paranoia, they proclaimed 'pretentious' as their defence, but the harbinger of grave disorder whose name might have been foretold two thousand years prior by the prophet of destruction knew more. The so-called 'wise man' (in such secular, embarrassing constructs of dipsomaniacal communion) had dismissed this triumph of revelation as a psychotic egomaniacal fantasy... the poor, geriatric fool... he knew nothing of the awesome truth by which our narrator mastered his apocalyptic verity.

No one knew... All men were but a sham and a dull collection of spherical cells by which they somehow (through some kind of interstellar genius) manifested consciousness. But what did the majority of this host of raven souls encourage as the basis of their sustenance? They captivated their evanescent purposes with a myriad of lascivious incarnations of ego, whereby each were a heroic master of the eternal gamete provider. This pathetic inculcation by moronic peers in adolescence, engineered via a primal philosophy, caused a destiny of saffron flames in all but the most strident of minds... he who controlled his essence with the most acute rectitude.

And so the fulgent minds exploded and roller coasted in their desperate attempts to cling to the wreckage of a society stooped in filth, but only a precious few wondrous beings could bypass the paradox of prevailing dissonance that paraded about society's collective consciousness like anathema. And these triumphant souls were to be the designers of the next world. The new reality.

And Princess Danni seemed suitable...

She wielded beauty. Her body was cut like perfect flesh that would one day be celebrated in statuesque form. Her naughty giggle expressed the joy of her being, and her insistence in her own mind that she was 'decent' manifested itself with an attitude that could garner the affections of the highest file of wise men.

She was… in conclusion… a hot chick.

So Prince Nicholas, as consumed with passion as he was, set about demonstrating quite why he was a suitable candidate for romance (that curious antidote to depression) in order to elucidate concisely exactly why Princess Danni was a femme (fatale?) of such breathtaking prestige.

Firstly, (although, in the precise gauging of a maiden's status, one could be forgiven for inaccurate sequencing of a belle's significance due to carefree hurling of locution from a cerebrally anarchic method), she was a potent character. Other broads, in their timorous cages, failed to convey the dynamic personality that Prince Nicholas sought in a potential matriarch, and Danni had those advantages in spades. (Indeed, often at times, betwixt the kaleidoscopic astral interchange of relayed mental imagery, Nicholas would muse upon what form of being a coalition of the two nuclei would manifest, should this delightful enchantress be the vessel of his progeny).

Secondly, (and do not dismiss this subsidiary point as inferior – one simply has to allocate definite placements of element in a tier based system to avoid confusion), she was formed from the branch of Aphrodite herself it seemed. Indeed, if Helen of Troy's face had launched a thousand ships, then Princess Danni was surely capable of setting forth a multitude of nautical vessels merely by batting an eyelid. Were her exceptional charisma and blistering pulchritude ever to be established officially as a visage and persona by which the mighty men of Blighty could guide their dreams? She could harness mighty power.

However, it was this latter point that had caused the aforementioned caustic whispers of the spirit to warn Prince Nicholas of her feelings. That she had, in her 'wrath' (for an unknown reason – ambiguity and assumption seemed to be the rudder by which the denizens of the locale steered their conjecture), sought to ruin the exalted being who held her in such high regard. Shattered for a moment to the crux by which our scribe emanated his reality, he sought to delineate exactly why this offensive information should be met with furrowed brows by all who understand justice.

It was a confusing period of existence for a plethora of souls, and such gleaned data from the psychic world reminded Nicholas of the Greek and Roman myths – the follies of bygone epochs whose nefarious methods dripped in ignorance and apparent delusion. Nicholas had long felt that due to his hallowed erudition that there was indeed, a divine entity – a higher intelligence – a supreme and mainly invisible deity to obey. The interpretation during days of yore to explain coherently this matter of heavenly awe had been met, however, time after time with vagaries, implausibility, and confusion. Indeed, Nicholas rarely explicated in the tavern the host of considerations and potential outcomes that he was party to, subscribed to a psychic mindset as he was, so he often masqueraded as the dupe, the fool (for he knew explaining the inexplicable was about as fruitful as declaring oneself immortal, prior to the end of time).

However, although his enlightenment was 100% factual and he had been granted a high rank by a number of disciples prior to the millennium, he knew the sins of England's subjects were manifold, and therein, was rarely surprised to find that a subordinate's callow idea might seek harm upon the innocent. Everyday, tales of horror paraded our eyes thanks to the media stream of this Orwellian wet dream, where the clutches of Satanic energy in the senses of asinine and wayward foe were disclosed to the populace as though it were elemental to our daily lives. Not only had that, but the swarm of imagery and euphonies emitting from a multitude of gizmos created a society of massively polarised agendas. He liked this, she liked that. He read this, she read that. He believed this was the best, she believed that was the best, etc. etc. Until, unless one acquiesced to the daily program of scheduled 'Big Brother' emissions as though it were a system of perfect knowledge, one could perceive beyond this onslaught of information, and find something so wondrous to celebrate about the triumph of the modern world. But perhaps denizens of planet Earth were becoming nonchalant and haughty in their assumption that this potentially transient era of techno wizardry would continue unabated?

Indeed, it would only take a few cells of indigenous partisans to a radical cause to muster massive change, should the intelligence, motive, and support be in place. The world had forever changed on that fateful day, when the Gemini stratosphere pierces were reduced to a bloody rubble by the bellicose insanity of a tiny brood of Allah hailing strategists operating under the guise as believers, and therein changed earth's fate (unless you concede to the concept that all is preordained anyway). So too, the subsequent incendiaries, whom brought terror to our turf, and the hilarity of crazed despots calling for the cull of the very people who grant them domiciles and prosperity. Thus, as all is causality, this created a massive cognitive network of rapidly alternating ideas and belief systems in a democratised system of the west, which are seeking methods by which to cope with such an alarming series of seditious events.

Thus, for a princess of the so called 'allies' to wish her admirer's essence to be quashed due to some undisclosed motive (no doubt stooped in a puerile quagmire of confused emotions) when he could help the occidental system maintain union and development in a number of ways, smacked of

LOVE IN THE PRISON OF PSYCHOSIS

darkness. And, being a mind gilded in light, darkness was the antithesis of Nicholas's whole agenda.

So... even when they labelled Prince Nicholas as 'psychotic', because they themselves knew not the latent and awesome power that some minds could exploit, and the now seemingly plausible truth of our writer being a telepath, the hidden truth of people's desires and thoughts were not always as hidden from him as others would wish.

He would wonder the streets, (he had a secret name that he told no one), and examine the metaphysical possibility that his theory on the spiritual versus the material was the totality of what he sought to explain as 'the higher truth'.

The theory went something like this... "The true thoughts of people's desires and opinions that they'd rather keep clandestine emerged in pockets of revelation when materialism was utilised, and therein expressed deeper truths about that person's veiled attitude and/or feelings". As adults, we disguise much of what we truly feel and think, due to societies insistence that we can't 'express our true beliefs', other than to loved and trusted ones, often for fear of being branded a moron. (Thus, reams and reams of effective information are prevented from being installed into others' minds due to the fact that we believe in our soul imprisonment that to expound one's true sentiments could result in situations too frightful to imagine).

This whole elaborate theatre we call society is thus a played out series of people interacting on the most fundamental (and often tedious) of levels, in order to harvest popularity and support, when all too often, it is simply an act of simpleminded vanity.

If the 'materialism is simply a physical embodiment that can often act as a cathexis by which we accidentally unleash a concealed personal attitude' is true, given that, most minds are shrouded in ignorance – then, perhaps the 'psychosis' they define Nicholas's state as being is in fact 'total actualisation and revelation' from a perspective of a far higher wisdom.

Of course, this whole study is still in its infancy, and I am still collating examples of what I precisely mean by this in order to fully convey exactly what it is I am attempting to demonstrate. Nevertheless, if all the borders and hindrances and mixed messages were removed from a person's mind, and he/she experienced mentality as powerfully as possible, and the capabilities it might possess... Could it not be argued that actually, Prince Nicholas did know things from a higher order, like that of the enlightened ones, and was not bound by temporal fixations of social cohesion in order to justify one's being as authentic, in part largely due to a predominance of fear in society?

LOVE IN THE PRISON OF PSYCHOSIS

He would, for now, leave the decision in Danni's mind... but she would never possess the right to cause an ill fate for one so rare. A swain of vast imagination may grant her some level of faux regal stature, but to actually act on such levels of imperial authority, without being officially recognised by the state was a potential offence in the golden corneas of Prince Nicholas. As such, these feelings should be discussed with depth, honesty and gravitas in order to come to know why she would dare even contain such a nefarious consideration in that effervescent soul.

Nicholas could not know for sure the direction to take, for no one really talked in depth at the water hole (attempt to discuss something of any true intellectual calibre, and be met with wide-eyed confusion and possible derision)... But he had seen the change in her state of mind, and, as such, sought to harvest that revolution of the grey matter, and induce a composition in order to finalise the fact that, although Nicholas wasn't perhaps the Messiah, he was actually 'an okay dude'. It seemed pertinent, therefore, that he should be met with approval by those with IQs higher than that of a fetid mollusc, or, indeed, half the population of planet Earth, and display his sincerity for her as an avatar of pure female goodness simply because:

1) He had nothing better to do.
2) No one else floated his boat.

3) It seemed like fun at the time.

Ergo, this triad of principles lay the cornerstone of action by which Nicholas pounded the ivories upon his console (that trusted friend), and reveal unto Princess Danni exactly the various solutions one might implement in order to benefit both parties mutually. (He had no need to be with a girl, should she not endear herself unto him. He was quite happy living the single existence for now). The fact that this love was not reciprocated was not the blemish in Nick's tapestry; indeed, he had long since known the emotional anguish associated with matters of affection, which was a primary justification for spending so many rotations of the sun without a partner. It was simply that he wished to convey unto the object of his desires, (which he declared to be the ultimate in the parochial region), the consideration that to be asked to escort this particular collection of animated matter was by no means a day to day event. Moreover, he simply sought the young Princess to remember this one particular individual for all time, creating a work that was designed for her, inspired by her, and focused entirely around her… for she was so special.

Now… I don't know what the widespread populace (of either gender) might make of such a gesture, but Nicholas felt it would be a suitable exercise, if only to do something 'different'. He considered that if he simply sat on his glutinous maximum all day regarding the television and receiving the constant barrage of drama, melodies, data and transitory glimpses of foreign humanoids, it would be a life wasted. A drone of the zone in his home on his own.

Verdict: An unacceptable stratagem to guide one's blessed gift of existence.

Solution: Do something... anything... that might have a positive effect on another embodiment of soul, which, in time, could engender all manner of developments in reality's wealthy series of conundrums and variables.

Thus... the keyboard was pounded with gusto as he mentally leapt upon his mighty steed, and galloped into the existential sunset leaving 'this' as the trace of a soul not fooled by the protocol of modernism. The stars in their trillions would continue to gleam within the infinite, and the earth would continue to spin about its axis. Yet, amid this bizarre panorama of personal existences, he would seek to throw a literary pebble in the mind-pool of a young female Padawan, so that she might develop with the passing of the seasons into a lady of utmost promise.

Producing ladies of unsurpassed social quality was a past time he had never truly considered, until that day he had seen her laugh. He knew the vision would be filed into his mental archive of 'cherished moments' until the day his last breath finally immersed itself into the wind; and his hearts final beat ceased the haemo-cadence of what was the embodiment 'Nicholas Clark'.

You might argue that such a humble moment in one's life is fairly paltry, given the wealth of experience we are subject to. Sure, it was not the LSD induced sense of feeling like a living God, or the series of epiphanies and revelations into the esoteric he'd been party to, or the moment his first love (Karen) agreed to be his girl... But the last half-decade had been such a pathetic and tedious series of uninspiring aspects of time – with little in the way of something truly magnificent to lay claim to – that amid this quarry of hours looking through a glass darkly, remembering you in that moment shone forth like a gemstone of promise.

Sure... it was corny... but no one else bothered to do this kind of shit. Everyone else capitulated to what was socially defined as 'the norm' (an illusion that didn't actually exist), and surrendered unto their own paranoia as nodes of a throng that were enslaved by their very own vanity and obsession. (See how controlled so many male 'sycophants to tribalism' were, moulded by a collective that utilised the kicking of air wrapped in fake leather around a garden as the prime source of much of their gratification). I would watch the hoards enter the public house dedicated to Solomon, and imagine how many of those men gazed upon your amazing countenance, and what manner of ungodly imaginings they kept hidden from public view. I can not say... but as a taciturn watcher of

LOVE IN THE PRISON OF PSYCHOSIS

this fatuous theatre we call culture, I would surmise a whole compendium of considerations that might lay before us all in time's oppressive onslaught.

Did I possess the basic in prophetic ability? What could I realise, whilst venerating you so, and penning these silly words? I place you on a pedestal not because I am a dreamer, (although it could be argued I am), but simply because it is entertaining for me to do so. Quintessential examples of female splendour are fairly rare in this modern world (often thanks to the system permitting all manner of heathens to engage in crimes of unlimited reproduction), and that fact, combined with a mind of definite intellect, is the cause throughout history of no end of men's actions. Even the wisest, the boldest, the richest men, have turned to fools in a second, simply to acquire the affections of a woman. This constant truism is a wonderful and rich source of most culture from any nation. (Ok, so in Roma, it's mainly tits and arse, whereas in China, it's all kung fu in the name of love and honour, and in America it's 'I KICK ASS, KISS ME'). But the essential ingredients of what creates a meaningful drama, or a reason for being, remains anchored to the foundations of that primal and ubiquitous urge for man and woman to unify. And the intricate complexity of each separate series of events, bound by conflict (whether physical, spiritual or emotional), is the basic nature of what formulates an entire race of homosapiens, each seeking their goals, to continue in aspiration.

So... in taking the time to place these predilections onto pulped wood, and send you a missive that I feel encapsulates just how honoured I am to have shared some brief moment of time with you, I feel that we have reached closure on a 'great perhaps' that never was to be. It is lamentable that, even in this circus of disparate ideologies, agendas, beliefs and coping mechanisms, whereby each person made flesh is an example of two minds coming together, unified by the forces of cross gender obsession, we cannot accept my advances as purely natural. The mockers might claim that it is my psychosis, the envious might use this as material to slander me in later years, and the ignorant might call me a 'twat' because I choose to express myself in such form. But no matter... I have delved deep into the very fabric of what constitutes mental existence, and I have analysed carefully what it is to be in possession of a mind and soul. I have spent long hours in my meditations attempting to compute and define what it is that exists. My findings are so far varying, and open to interpretation. Yet amid this flurry of firing synapses and sparkling neurons, and however much I try to focus on the arts and sciences, (both two noble pursuits that augment my *raison d'etre*), I remain a man who desires love on occasion (as foolish as that sounds). To consequently assert those sensations (and a woman like you would produce those feelings in most men, were they bold enough to admit their inherent feelings), I consider my actions authentic, and it is regrettable that such florid and unique approaches have fallen on stony ground. Were it not for the strength of the truths that compound my entirety through time and space, where I have gazed upon the miraculous, I might be forgiven for taking a razor, and slicing my throat.

But this would be fundamentally stupid, as I am still very much pleased to exist on this inter galactic orb in the middle of vast nothingness, albeit one full of rather moribund examples of human imagination. So don't worry about that, old girl. Suffice to say, I shall go forth, and continue to seek what I might find, (in accordance with the codex), and enjoy those quiet moments to myself when I imagine collating all of the actual thoughts of those I know (were we to know such thoughts), into a computer. And then process an algorithm that calculated the precise actions each individual must undertake in order to fulfil their lives to the level they aspire to. Were such a concept possible, it might be interesting to then program into the equation a system by which the DNA of each member of my reality, (all those I know are 'members of my reality'), is deconstructed so that the most suitable pairing for procreation is simulated. (I am now rambling about something that is irrelevant to the point in hand, and am imagining what the offspring of Rod and Eve might be like – so I will cease).

Given that I believe there is a definite likelihood for there are to be more than five dimensions to the universe, and that I have already squandered enough time seeking to know you, I shall henceforth keep you in my dreams. I will keep the image of you forever, and the grace you brandished (as though it were typical for all natives to retain such wonder), and smile in retrospect whenever I am mentally desolate, for I was blessed to meet you.

If I have caused you harassment, I apologise... it was not my intention. I therefore ask you to forgive me for my all too human stupidity in yearning for one as excellent as 'you' to be my girl, and hereby rescind my previous attempts to woo thee. I hope that any mental discomfort I have propagated in your mind is hereby repaired, and that any concerns you have that I might be:

a) Sociopath
b) Perverted
c) Obsessed
d) A twat

Are hereby proven to be without evidence and that the only invective or defamation that is so far plausible when dispelling my nature as invalid is along the lines of:

a) Doesn't he go on a bit?
b) Oh, I'd wish he'd shut up, and let someone else get a word in.

LOVE IN THE PRISON OF PSYCHOSIS

c) He drinks and smokes too much.
d) I wonder if he's on drugs.

The latter is a moot point, admittedly, but I feel that my entire philosophy in life has been radically altered by my usage of narcotics in the past, and that is one reason, perhaps, that I am either:

a) Mentally deranged. (I don't believe a mentally deranged person would have gone for as long as I have without being sectioned – do you?).
b) That I really have expanded my mind into supreme areas of enhanced insight.

Anyway... As Yoda once said 'the dark side is quicker, visually more seductive', and there you have the glamorous attributes of a whole social system based on the host of imagery we have bombarding our corneas every day.
"Give them what they want, and they will follow you". One notorious axiom of maintaining people's loyalty. Also... when done by mortals... first rule of a society destined to sink to the lowest common denominator of perversion, greed, vanity and gossip. Civilisation teeters on the edge of the next phase of humanities revelation, but where will you be when I think of you?

It is written, 'the first shall be last, and the last shall be first'. One interpretation of this is that all those deemed as winners in the modern world will be damned as conspirators and agents of the evil Empire, come a possible revolution. (If one believes in a revolution of some sort, occurring at any given time in the future; not that 'I am a communist, who believes Marx is always right, and that revolution is the key').

Here endeth the inaugural episode of Prince Nicholas's treatise, whose candid approach to this world of trickery rewards him both major respect, and plenty of disdain.

Second sight.

I saw you again last night... working on a Saturday night at the saloon of King David, and I tried not to stare at you. We talked for a moment about your first two weeks at University, and it concerned me that you weren't a happy lass. Every time you spoke, I saw those glistening eyes beaming their effeminate marvel, and every smile you granted me was like a portal to the dreams of legends. You don't only take my breath away, you practically encourage asthma. I have to smoke cigarettes and drink lager if only to dampen the soaring affections I have coursing through my veins, but they do not become dampened. They increase in agape ecstasy, and my whole being shines in your presence as though I am a divine entity, but only I feel it. I mask the endless things I would like to talk to you about, were we ever to actually go out for a time, and simply accede to the course of dialogue you direct.

LOVE IN THE PRISON OF PSYCHOSIS

I sense all the energy of existence around me, and hear the multitude of voices of the clientele in its cacophonic babble, but one glimpse of your sensational being, and the voices deteriorate into a distant void of extraneous nonsense. Only you, the principle cathexis of that locality beckon my every spiral of the mind, and I hate myself for being so pathetic that you do not want to know me. I know in the past I have been a little extreme for the rather stifled tastes (and let's admit it, boring bastards) of much of the indigenous populace, but I cannot deny the intensity of my existence. I must be unleashed at least on some level, rather than timidly sitting in a self imposed delusion that I am mature and 'wise'. I weave these words about your mind as a desire to communion, and for the simple fact that it pleases me to mine the soul for deeper meaning in matters of the heart, rather than utilise the Neanderthal efforts of other mortal men, such as 'Fancy a shag, love?'

However, at the same time, I feel a bit like a prick writing these words... I mean 'it's all a bit gay', possibly... all lovey dovey clap trap... but Shakespeare rocked my world at school for a time, and it is out of reverence to his world changing methods that I doff my cap to his legacy. I seek to convey exactly what it is that flourishes about my entity when I look at you, and hear those delicate vocal timbres emanate from your mouth. The maxim 'You... rock... my... world...' circulates within my evanescent skull as I feel my pupils expand as they seek to encompass the sheer splendour you espouse. I am determined to make you matter in an ocean of souls all prevaricating about the core of reality's substance. Six billion minds, all randomly wondering upon the surface of this globe, and you and me, amid these phenomena, have met via the passage of existence. This prodigious fact is combined with the point that really, as I study the contours and shadows of my stupid face in the reflection of my monitor, my mind's eye contains too often an image of you. In thousands of years of human reproduction, you and I have collided in a seemingly irrelevant zone, and we have shared the motions of the eons as they dance their shimmering majesty. Danni... who'd have thought it? Where were you conceived? What are you inner thoughts? What is your destiny? Who was your first love? What have been the triumphs of your life so far? What are your fears? What do you desire in life most?

I quash the obsession for a moment in order to engage in a sense of logic that might teach me which route to take at this bifurcation of fate. Do I allow you to read this, when it is really just the notional meandering of a man captivated, (the age old situation), or do I keep it from your view, so that it will never fall into the wrong hands? Such a sincere exploration of my own heart is met with potential suffering should I fall too deep into the morass of emotion, so I maintain equanimity where possible, although the gravitational pull of

LOVE IN THE PRISON OF PSYCHOSIS

your lustrous soul is too much to resist at some junction of the deeper motives.

Shiiiiiiit…

The tenebrous destiny I often fear manifests once again in the nadir of my imagination. The mental activity and seemingly telepathic intimacy with the spirits taunt me and challenge my sanity… I anchor logic and reason as the two prime foundations by which to maintain peace of mind, but the anarchic pull of 'the extra sensory perception' shatters my dreams into a million useless bits of information, a ravaged cornucopia of distraught loss and failure. I engineer a soul enhancement, a wind of faith billows through my being, the only solution to the occasional collapse of rationalism. I insist that I am in charge of my destiny, however much the contemptuous phantoms seek to wreck my optimism, and I generate energy pulses through every nerve to combat the concept of nihilism and negativity.
There is more than nothing… Nihilism is a non sequitur, yet people's insistence that they are in possession of the facts about the state of things when I know they are not causes me some resentment on occasion, but I remember my illumination, and thereby seek to enhance my existence. Does this all sound vague? Does this all smack of a young man attempting to explain the absolute? Scientists talk of quantum energy; artists talk of 'beauty is truth'; musicians talk of harmonies and choruses; generals talk of war, and

politicians talk of law. But I wish to encompass all that it is to be a human, and go further than this... beyond borders... Into the grand expanse of the ambiguous, subconscious, swamp of the million dollar questions... the questions that still none can answer, and perhaps discover throughout my entire time one revelation about life that provides people with illumination.

Deeper I go, deeper into the abysm of cognition, where acumen serves as a valiant ally, and peer for sustained periods of time into the neo-cortex's dormant capabilities to manage the vast streams of information that volley amid its pseudo-holistic channelling. A biological device so drenched in potentiality that were a host of neophytes to be augmented with wise indoctrination to the contemporary divination, this purposely designed facet of humanity would expand into the higher dimensions. Once this might occur, man and woman alike might see the infinite nature of expanded consciousness, where their specific entities are all pieces of an elaborate historical mosaic of dreams, thoughts, beliefs, ideas and imaginations. To shimmer in the apex of pathos, visions pounding my cerebral vista, I can conceive of the almighty as an actuality that is but a whisper away, and beyond that frontier, which harbours the dichotomy between logic and the supernatural, resides the glory of the ancient of days. To know this is to know the absolute, and to know the absolute is to be a master of existence. The subjects in my reality appear as strangers I seek to comprehend, but only you have opened the

LOVE IN THE PRISON OF PSYCHOSIS

portal to my warmest affections, and therein, I am caught in an enigma. Will she ever be surpassed by another, who might actually covet me as I crave her? I know that I will not marry unless I am bonded with a female who is exceptional, and that I can trust myself not to betray due to feelings of her being inadequate at some level. For this woman I speak of (who might not exist) to exceed the wonders you harness, she would have to be so sublime that I'm not even certain if creation can provide such a prototype. So I dwell in mental solitude, waiting for a partner who might be acceptable, and not conjoin with any old woman who might grant me a loving smile. And as the passing of the seasons persists relentlessly, time itself authoring me only a fraction of its monumental expanse, my presence on this planet only ever lessens in duration. As such, I patiently await what experiences of pleasure I might carve from this mass of atomic interplay, and continue tirelessly to stake my claim within the social matrix of multifarious thought processes. Fabricating from the heart of what I am a series of literary promulgations by which I declare the zenith of my current state of mind, I divulge this news unto only the very treasured. I allow the console by which I generate new realities to accept every tapping of the keys so that I might consolidate the mind merger I scheme, and therein coalesce this short mass of utterances unto your mind. The outcome of such an action cannot be known at this juncture, but I await with intensifying curiosity as to what your tender brain might make of such a sprawl of terms. You might think me prolix or abstruse, but I seek to summarise a whole swarm of sentiments and explain evidently the whole of love from a foolish male's perspective. It may seem trite, and prosaic in places, but playing with words, and expressing my honest feelings is an act by which I practise constantly. Hence... I seek to explain the totality of what it is to adore, and I trust you will appreciate that men cannot help what they sometimes feel.

Do not worry though; I am not a crazy person (although others might beg to differ). I simply believe that love is an essential ingredient in life's rich voyage of the stimuli, and although that devotion to a cause is prevalent ubiquitously, it happens to be YOU who found herself at the axis of my personal fondness (the probability of which should stagger you, not repulse you).

Never mind... I understand that I am inadequate as a beau for a number of reasons, and as such, will not pester you, but simply banish this series of lyrical outbursts to a moment in history. However, I can at least say I 'had a go', rather than hide my feelings and remain confined to a cowardly status of 'if only I asked', which is the regrettable folly of many a timid man's remorse.

So I register this tirade within your heart, and expect little in the way of recompense, other than the knowledge someone like you is present in the active principle of existence. I crank the tunes, sip

LOVE IN THE PRISON OF PSYCHOSIS

a tea, drag on a Marlboro, and allow the mellifluous recollections of the snippets of chronology that garnered me your transient favour to make molten my soul. My every breath evaporates in sequence into the atmosphere, swirling the molecules contained within, and the grand supposition that man is generally a benevolent entity causes me to muse on the higher plains of what might be. The church of the poisoned mind is my sanctuary, and I prepare the altar in repentance, for I damaged myself. The euhemerism of the present mythology is rife with great men, and I don't know where I come on the scale of worth. However, knowing that for a time I was celebrated by some causes me to settle into a gentle slumber of hope, with the consideration that my soul is not without meaning (if any are)…

Time lapse – unknown chronology.

I dwell in the soul wrecking absolution of the heightened mind hell bent on finding worth in an array of limited and ambiguous mortals all seeking meaning in a diverse construct of multifarious suppositions. I quell the damning voices on the wind seeking to subdue my spirit of fortitude, and long for the days of yore, when we laughed in splendour whilst educated at prestigious mansions of higher discipline.
Oh… Danni… How you'd have enjoyed our ideology in that temple to adolescent conditioning… but now reality smacks of a whole host of raven agendas propounded by less than

adequate mortals each seeking to placate the multitude of detractors via a vainly endorsed method of simple double think. (I was told to stop talking bullshit in the pub years ago when I mentioned 'double think'. Problem is... the scaly who derided me for such a term was not aware of the potent influence of Orwell within our contemporary sociological dynamic).

Anyway... it is not of issue... as my mind scurries and expands and spins in a number of directions, I choose you as an apex of decency by which I anchor my raging rapids of emotive free thought. You have caused a great tsunami of motives to eddy out of control. I seek to salvage some of this maelstrom of passion (and am reminded of a book we read at prep school), but I cannot muster the definite providence by which I can wipe you from my memory banks. You are... in potentiality... the ultimate, and I kneel to your inherent wonder. (Jeesh...).

With Love,

Nick.

END OF LETTER

I suppose you probably think I'm a twat... Writing all of that. But writing is my only permitted escape from this prison. I don't plan to let her read the

LOVE IN THE PRISON OF PSYCHOSIS

letter necessarily. It is a personal exploration of my own heart over a woman I know will probably not wish to be with me. I simply wrote it to quell the tide of boredom that the screws insist on applying to my one definite chance at existence. So I keep it stored on file, with all my other dreams, so that maybe one day, in the future, when the prison is liberated by some higher revelation, my words of love might be registered in at least one brain.

(In truth, I have already implanted the letter as a vague memory into one of my mind control executives, so that she might realise my schizophrenia is not insanity, but an aspect of expanded consciousness. I have this young woman see me in my luxurious cell once a fortnight to analyse and run tests on my thought process. If she doesn't like a thought, she seeks to remove it from my mind using vocal mind alteration techniques. Thankfully, the prison electronics department isn't yet at a level whereby all our inner thoughts can be seen and screened on the national broadcast facilities. When that happens, we could be facing some such horror the likes of which not even Eric Blair considered).

I need to venture out now, into the commerce sector... I'll be back in half an hour. I need to transpose some freedom credits from one account to another. I don't have much. Just enough to buy cigarettes to help kill myself, and a small subscription to the 'cyber-portal of manufactured thought control', but at least I can look at inhabitants of the prison while in the commerce sector and think 'I'm better looking than 71.342% of you unsightly strangers".

RETURN OF THE LIGHT RIDER

I'm back... its grey out there... English grey... For months on end we have that kind of overcast cloud coverage, and yet some still believe we live in the greatest country on the planet. What poppycock. It's like the first cycle of hell in the city today. (The city is the Central Processing Unit Commerce Sector for a local province). The inmates looked grim as usual. The winter chill is hugging at their projections for the coming periods... We're on the brink of half a year of typical drudgery. The voices were telling me that my first love had been murdered, and that my mother had been sodomised by a group of BNP members, because they thought I was left wing. The BNP are worse than the screws... at least the screws have principles. The principles of the BNP are the 'way of the demons'. They often move in groups of at least three or four, and their minds are pure venom. What they don't appreciate is that if they think they're the superior race, then the superior race is an ugly, stupid, violent, drunken set of working class bastards who can't string an intelligent sentence together, and actually have no qualms in taking a young girl's life, or raping an innocent boy's mother.

LOVE IN THE PRISON OF PSYCHOSIS

Hmmm... I'm not so sure that's my idea of the master race. Don't know about you. I think the elitist camps spawned a far better breed of man. Erudite, trained, lucid, generally better groomed, able to make money on the whole, from a good gene pool, often pleasant and polite. What do I know though? My training at an elitist camp mainly involved laughing a lot in heaven with my brothers on dope. We didn't much care for the privilege at the time. We thought we were in a concentration camp for rich boys... and in a way, we were, but by God, it was better than the real prison. The prison of human scum that we constantly have to suffer.

Hiding from trouble, witnessing rage and violence and drunkenness as the inhabitants lose control due to their improper mental development. I dream of an Exodus to a utopian Island in the sun (possibly Mauritius), where my friends and family can enjoy each day in warmth, peace and good fun. But I know from experience that utopia chasing can often end up leading to quite the opposite. I just take each day as I find it now. I'm glad I can still walk and breathe, and communicate with simpletons on a very mundane level, but I'm just passing the time until I'm dead. Don't get me wrong. I don't really want to die, but if this is it (and I know there is more), and the totalitarian greyness of the prison is all I have to look forward to, living without a beautiful girl, or the high of dope... then... well... time will be my cell too.

Jeesh. Even the fourth dimension is a prison now. I used to hide my dreams in my neo cortex, knowing I had time to play in them, but if they amount to nothing but a few synapses glowing, just like all the other matrix dwellers... Big deal. I'm just an embodiment of cells like any living being on this planet. I'm animated, and can generate mental processes, but if I'm not state endorsed (which I doubt they'll want, considering the nature of these dark times), then my enlightenment counts for nothing but a personal insight, when rightly, it should muster glory in a team of millions. I can rejoice in my cell all I like, lying on my bed, staring at the ceiling – alone – thinking: 'I know there is more to this life'... but if others aren't aware of it, and others don't believe it... Then what good is it to mankind?

There were so many ugly people in the CPUCS today... so many poor examples of breeding. So many results of a drunken shag in the ghettos and slums. So many offensive examples of human reproduction. I was ashamed to be a part of Beth's island for a while. Then I had to open the door for a BNP street shock team. I once had a dream that my deceased grandfather (whose death I accidentally caused) came back to me with a green moustache, and told me that 'when I grow up, I'll be a doorman'. Maybe he was right. My job is a joke, and all I do when out is hold doors open for people. I wish I could be a doorman, but for the 'doors of perception'. Take people out of this prison and grant them their wishes, like a genie. However, I am regulated and relegated to the position of a psycho, because the system won't condone my philosophy of 'cosmic free thought'. People don't like it, they don't get it. They stick to their own little ways, like discussing the latest soap opera, or listening to a rubbish tune on the prison airwaves and thinking it's great. I lament this sorry zeitgeist of phoneys pretending they're living in a better prison than other nations... Like Burma, which really is the pits. Yet the threats and mental torturing they place me under is tantamount to a new wave terror. A new wave denizen inspired attempt at solution finding ever since the September 11th micro apocalypse. Causality... Damn causality... The reason for reactions... Do this, and get that. Didn't those Muslim terrorists even think what they might be creating on that day? Did they consider the repercussions? The sun went out for New York then, and the world was plunged into more of a terror than usual. For what? Envy? Arrogance? Evil? Hatred? I can't think of many similes that one can associate with the collapse of the twin towers that suggest it was something positive, other than damnable rage of disturbing theology generated in the zealous aortas of a bevy of ill disciplined hell raisers. As for it being a spiritual event... well... either they were demented angels of God's wrath (which they probably thought they were), or they were simply psychotic, and I didn't see the faces of angels on the mug shots, not the shimmering wings and sparkling halos. I saw menace...

I meander... The events of that day were extraordinary, but it's only impinged on the world as a whole… The prison is a darker place now, all over the world. Inhabitants still attempt to have fun, and escape the chains of mortal responsibility, but everything is graver now… Suspicious eyes scan you in the tunnels. Every Asian gets considered internally as a suspect for a crime yet to be committed. No one can be sure whom to trust. The freedom the west sought has collapsed into an immoral pool of secrets and lies, creating the prison of conscience partly through thoughtless transgression and self imposed means to present oneself as decent, when in their heart of hearts, they are anything but. This is the truth as I subscribe to it, knowing that the voices I hear tell me of the coming drama, the events that might transpire in order that retribution and a grim form of justice are paraded about society as a warning of the word 'freedom' being utilised as a euphemism for 'Satan's playground'. We've let the devil in… We've all let the devil in… and now he's manifesting in our fears and dreams, and like a tempestuous phantom of crazy immorality, he seeks dominion over the souls that grant his methods as intelligent. They're growing in number. First it was hundreds, then thousands… Then it will be tens of thousands, and then hundreds of thousands. I use the term 'Satan' as a traditional concept to describe an overall collective psychological reaction to various belief systems that appear inadequate to a fairly intelligent person. Evil is an esoteric mental corruption of honour and faith. You can see it in the eyes of a few people sometimes – the longing to be

LOVE IN THE PRISON OF PSYCHOSIS

terrible... Their eyes glow and that knowing smile creeps upon their visage like a representation of the omnipresent demonic sense as hope. That's the trick with the dark side... it seeks to pretend it's wiser. It seeks to pretend it knows all things, when in fact; it is often a madness that has overrun the psyche masquerading as a higher knowledge.

I need a drink. The depression of another day of threats, greyness and solitude has begun to claw at my very fibre, and a meditation in my sleeping quarters with a cup of tea and a cigarette will be just the remedy to administer a little spice.

That's better... I've got a little lift. I've just spoken to one of my oldest brethren from the elitist training academy. He's stationed up in Glasgow, in the slums. His name is Putz, and he's a great guy. We have been close friends for fifteen years... and we've never once fallen out. He's too cool to fall out with. You can't help but love the guy. Handsome, funny, brave, crazy, cool... but he's been married and divorced to a female inmate before I've even got married. No woman would want me... That's the problem. I'm too warped, and my sexual ability is probably inadequate. Furthermore, a lady of merit would assume some level of freedom credits in order to enhance her assumptions of importance. I would love to be able to garner the kind of zeros on my account balance that would entice the female of my dreams... but alas, my past with the bohemian renegade tribes and my ineptitude at working in a typical slave job ensure I remain *skint*. I had a girlfriend recently, who was pretty good looking, but she was a bitch. I dumped her because she lied, and I felt my blood turn to ice as she went out for a meal with her ex. (Who happened to be a love crazed Islamist).

So... I dumped her by text message. Not very gallant, for sure... You're probably screaming at me now saying 'you bastard!' I don't wish to be treated like that though. Her ex boyfriend kept sending her perverted texts during our brief relationship. He was still insanely passionate about her and hated the ground I walked on for grabbing her out of time. She had M.E, and although one morning she said that I was 'the best sex she'd ever had' (no doubt a total lie), she was hard work... I can't trust modern women... Too scheming and liberated. They're the chink in my armour whenever I am dating. If I were a successful man, who was wielding a ten-inch phallus, then maybe I would be a little less insecure when it comes to relationships... but I'm neither. I'm a psychotic who hears demons and angels, and walks the prison passageways thinking about a ninja in white I call 'Snowflake'. He is my guardian angel, I like to think, and prevents true crimes being committed against me – because he's wise, spiritual, and quicker in a fight than Jackie Chan. But I am not Snowflake... he is my astral protector... the hero dormant in my soul.

LOVE IN THE PRISON OF PSYCHOSIS

And so I return to the locus of freedom credit transactions, where I am paid pittance to sit in a seat waiting for the rare event of a person to enter the shop and purchase a mind control sequence. (Why do you think TV programs are called 'programs'? They 'program' you). For the expenditure of £3.50, they can absorb, on average, two hours of carefully filmed footage by a host of multifarious filmmakers and be taken on a celluloid trip into another person's vision. These films have in the main cost millions of dollars/pounds to create, and half the time, people sit there for two hours, and at the end think 'that was crap'. Such is the way of prison life. On occasion, a film will be so effective at suspending someone's disbelief and taking them on a fantastic mind voyage, that the whole world will generate a frisson of delight, and, in a few exceptional cases, they will radically change culture on a macro level. This is the joy of film – escapism. Like TV, or religion, billions of people are glued to the TV screens on a daily basis being transported to places of fiction. Stories written by intelligent minds, inspired often by something real, but extrapolated and enhanced exponentially to a far altered final product that will either fly or falter depending on the audience response. The society of the spectacle is prevalent, and yet people dismiss drug users as 'escaping from reality'. What hypocrisy! How can they slander a toker from enjoying what they consider to be 'enhancement', rather than an escape, and then go and watch 'Lord of the rings' and say 'oh, how wonderful'. To the right minds when under the influence of the sacred herb, "Lord of the Rings" seems pretty naïve and childish. Then to be told by a government that celebrates this series of fantasies we are not allowed to 'escape' in a truly powerful way is appalling. Renegade inmates do it anyway... millions of them. Very few of them dying.

But no... Because I smoked cannabis everyday for 3 years, and started to hear voices, (for reasons which could be numerous, other than blaming the drug alone) they now damn me if I ever wish to enter Cloud 9000 and giggle in the empyrean realms of deep beauty.

I blame the rock and rave scene for a lot of this excessive drug use. Not that I'm deriding their behaviour. I can totally understand it, but societies massive dichotomy of philosophy over the drug issue is now so omnipresent that we only hear a one sided view from the prison authorities. On the tanoy system we hear how bad drugs are for you, when huge numbers of people in the media are using them for some of the very ideas sober people champion. Why don't we hear on the news?

"Today, Simon Jameson took LSD, and realised that the universe was an infinite utopian aspect of divinity whose conceptualisation was of an intelligence far beyond that of us mere mortals, and how the power of love will vibrate through the gargantuan levels of molecules for all time as a positive energy stream"?

Wouldn't that be interesting? But no... Bias, one sided arguments fail to tell people the whole truth about smoking a joint. Ok, so maybe it can, in a few cases, lead to mental health issues. Then again, you're not likely to feel too well if you drink 8 pints a day, everyday, for twenty years – but it happens, and most people accept moderation as a reasonable balance to guide one's life by.

Not only that... but classing cannabis as an illegal drug is one reason people go onto harder stuff. If people were allowed to smoke dope legitimately, then people would be more trusting of a government, which prohibits 'Heroin', which can really destroy lives. The fact that a government has prohibited cannabis creates two scenarios – equally erroneous:

1) Many people believe cannabis is a wicked thing to smoke, and in their ignorance, judge and deride those who try it.
2) Those who *do* try it, often have a great time, laugh a lot, feel beautiful and special, and think "my goodness... If they're making something that makes me feel this great illegal, I wonder how cool the stronger stuff is".

Hence, this is why people will tend to experiment with harder drugs, because their experience with cannabis for the first time can be so enthralling, that they disrespect a government policy that prevents such a wondrous sensation from taking place, and thus ignore the warnings of everyone in the prison, because we're all conditioned to believe everything said by the media thought control system is entirely accurate and based on deep knowledge.

Cobblers...

Anyway... My trip about my mind has reverted back to my desire to enter the 'ultra realm' again, and take a ride on the interstellar mind expansion love carousel of psychoactive uber bliss. I must return to the point in hand... and that is... why am I writing all this? I want to be with Danni, but the system doesn't tolerate relationships that are deemed unsuitable due to onerous factors. I see the misery in so many faces, and yet I see the joy in Danni's. She doesn't mind the prison. For someone her age, she wields a lot of influence as a peer to her age group in the local area (which, admittedly, is 11 years younger than me). She's only 19, but by heck, she's well crafted. I cannot concentrate on my studies while I know I have had my advances rejected by her. Nothing matters in the prison much anymore other than to get bored, sit in obedience, not start any trouble, and have a few lagers at night for self-serving exhilaration. The local commerce centre is full of drugs, apparently... but they keep discreet. I can't do them anyway, or I'll be homeless. Homeless in the prison island is about as bad as you can get. At least the cells have warmth and entertainment. Being a vagabond thrown to the pavements to scavenge for food is the lowest of the low. The sheer nadir of social status. I'd last ten minutes on the streets... I'd be back on drugs in no time, in order to cope... but it wouldn't be coping. It would no doubt hinder matters, and I'd be in the gutters in my rags looking up at the heavens knowing that there was now no future rank of prison status that I could possibly ascribe to, given the appalling situation. So here I am... stationed in 'DVD mind control department' giving out mainly boring films to people who need something to fill a gap in their lives. I am the gap filler... I fill those empty pockets of down time people need, so they don't have to sink too far into their own realities, but reach out into the stories of others to develop their ideas of the cultural design.

Thus, the matrix is made ever more complicated.

My mind glows as I pen these words. The locution streams from my brain like a motorway of cars at night... each incandescent red, white and yellow beam a glimmering idea interweaving at varying speeds along the speedway of consciousness... my mental emissions scatter upon the wood pulp, and I declare I am penning the words of a tome that will linger in the minds of a few for years to come. These are the lessons of the psychedelic warrior of the infinite dimensions...whose ultra fantastic experiences of holistic mind prism 'spectrum running' have formed a unique mind in a world of nodes. I delve into the primordial soup of human thought, and consider what my objective is in this populace. There are billions of women out there... Billions... and I rarely get fancied by any of them. Am I so appalling to the mind of a female? Why can't I win Danni's fair hand? I must leave it to the cosmic order of things... I must accept fate's lessons, and if I am to be joined with that wondrous creature, which keeps me dreaming, it will be inscribed in the annals of time's punishing flow.

I had to break concentration for a moment there... A prisoner came in, and asked for a film that 'didn't require much thought'. A lot of people don't like to think too much... it scares them. I'm exactly the opposite... I love to think. I love to use my brain to its maximal potential and endeavour to explain the reasons for my epiphanies. I love to philosophise on what it is that constitutes decent cogency. I try to second-guess society... I try to understand the macro-vision... I try to foresee the next 'big fad' that will emerge from the brain of a bright spark, and take the inmates into another little buzz of obsession.

Johnathon Livingstone Seagull pops up in my brain as the bird that sought freedom... I never liked the book when I first read it. I thought it dumb. Now I appreciate its simplicity and idealistic innocence. It appeals to the masses, which seek simplicity in the face of gross technological and intellectual complexity. However, I decree this as a denial of the reality, and one's own honed potentiality. The anthropomorphism still seems twee, but I have come to accept that the varying opinions of minds from all walks of life find their solace from the pain of incarceration in all manner of diverse literature. I wish I could take you somewhere... Somewhere better than tedium. Somewhere higher than the Sun, to a new galaxy where we feel like fulgent Gods of the universe, ready to solve every intergalactic crisis with our dormant super powers we neglect to appreciate we might possess. I long for a Diaspora to heaven, where the angels fly about our souls like golden supermen, granting us all the knowledge of the divine... but as I have said before... the holy codex's we have granted to us by the prophets are so utterly ineffective at producing a decent and workable theology to grasp, that we falter at every separate dream.

So I cling to this moment in my existence. 5:59pm Tuesday 18th October 2005. A day and a half has passed since I began writing this letter. The system knows nothing of it yet, but I wonder what it will make of it? Will it be censored and destroyed? Or will it be produced so that others can linger for a moment in the mind of a stranger who is reaching out to others as a last vain attempt to make them know the prodigious incarnation that is our embodiments, and how we mollify to tedious logic and system regulations when we could shine like immortals in the valleys of Elysium. Where every blessed soul communes to build a city of true vision that shines a light of hope throughout the globe. A city forged from gold and gems and quantum intelligence. Where every inhabitant is a master in their own right, and crime is a forgotten social malediction. Where stupid beliefs are seen for what they are, and we at last have a sentient glimpse into the wonder of the infinite; and live long lives of laughter and brilliance as the joyous music pours from every sound system installed into its many crevices. Where we become like angels ourselves, of our own earthly paradise, no longer contaminated by the inadequacies of ancestors, or the folly of diverse belief systems based on metaphysical and unproven notions. Where we can laugh at the history of man, who fought battles over forces they couldn't understand, and where we are allowed to get high on narcotics as a reasoned aspect of man's need to expand their consciousness from a sociological perspective, rather than an oppressed dream that seems so distant and is wrongly labelled criminal thanks to the over excesses of some immoral curs.

Sure... it's a dream. It's a fairytale based on already established ideas. It's antithesis to dystopia... but why shouldn't it be a reality for some at one point in the future? Why does people's cynicism in the prison capitulate to a ruling body that insists we must behave the way we are told, and yet have never managed to stamp out the dark horrors of crime and evils? To dream... perhaps... *is* the dream... At least the prison allows us that much freedom. Sure... it's in the minds, but maybe that is the best place for them. Maybe that's the idea of the system... to create a dreamscape. A vast and elaborate warren of families all living in a utopian fantasy, formed largely from the editing and manipulation of images, sound and text on the TV and in writing. It's a novel conceit... I admit... masquerading as a perfect human to the audiences of millions, while in the quiet moments of your own actual life, you are a torrent of misdemeanours. What a design for life... A multilayered fabrication of data to imply a system of perfection that, at ground level, simply is not workable. Thus, a conflict arises... and in that conflict, it becomes a game. But a very serious game... and one you don't want to lose. Goodies and baddies... Exactly what the Hollywood propaganda system has been seeking to make the world believe in for years. The idea of the archetypical 'hero' (with his moral boons and courageous selflessness) verses the 'villain', the symbolic archetype of all the human characteristics the writer seeks to banish from his own latent darkness. It creates a schizoid culture... every writer enhancing the good, and punishing the bad in their own psyches. The moral codes in him are gauged though... but how, and why? Why does he think a certain characteristic is good, and another is bad? Is he trained in the ways of the religious masters? If the American hero's we see populating our screens were all heroes like the idea of Christ, then there wouldn't be one shot fired. What is the body count emanating from imagination over the last 60 years on the silver screen? It must be huge… how many blanks have been fired in replica guns to symbolise the power of the righteous over that of the wicked? How many millions of fans have longed to be a dark anti-hero, on a crusade to change the world?

Many… but society have become absolutely drenched in this clichéd and fundamental approximations of narrative. This is why I am writing this letter to you, my friend, so that you can know for certain that the concept of 'enlightenment' is true, and does exist. That there is a divine realm of genius wonder and beauty, but you must be strident in your rectitude to gain the crown. Stick to your own mind… and garnish it with the ancient and modern wisdom's you *do* rationalise and comprehend, and do not submit to those moral codes and ideas you cannot fathom, because that will simply cause you dissonance and paranoia. Take charge of the miraculous incarnation of spirit that is YOU, and do not be persuaded by zealous men who charm their way into your minds, but leave it furnished with confusion and stupidity. Ignore the hatred of people, and know that even if the world hates you, the divinity does not. Don't subscribe to foolish tribal mentalities, when such mentalities are based largely on geography, or place of birth, or family heritage, if it doesn't seem correct to you. It is folly to follow the crowd like lemmings over the cliff.

LOVE IN THE PRISON OF PSYCHOSIS

Enlighten yourself in your preferred way, and do not yield to the horrors of a concept as monstrous as hell through cowardice, thereby becoming a fool in the eyes of many. Do good on your own terms, so that you might feel heroic as time passes, and you are still granted the freedom to wonder the corridors of the luxurious prison, and not find yourself incarcerated in maximum security due to blatant idiocy. The world is not perfect... do not think it is... so start a cause, however small, that is based in positivism... Grab life by the essence of your own power, and don't squander that power, and find yourself in trouble by others with more freedom credits. Ignore the cynicism of people who deny your ideas, and know that an idea is only an idea until work and effort has been applied to it in order for it to grow. Should that idea be good enough, it might grow to levels you couldn't even imagine, taking you places you'd never thought possible, and perhaps, if you're extremely lucky, grant you enough freedom credits to win a mansion in Olympus. Don't envy the rich though; money does not bring all things. A man could pay me £50 billion, and I still would not be able to grant him enlightenment from the divine realms... And yet, I am in debt, on £5 an hour, and I possess that treasured apotheosis of illumination.

If you are born into low status housing areas, seek to change it for the better. Don't just accept it as your lot, or wait for someone else to make it all better... Conjure your own ideas to improve matters, and bring other people on board where possible. Get inspired, get light, and follow the path to your destiny faithfully with fortitude. Never quit on something you are passionate about, for even the slightest attempt at something creative or intelligent will lay a corner stone in your own history for you to enjoy again later in life as you reflect on the good you did.

Don't presume, if you believe in the bible, that we are living in the last days. We might be, but people have been saying this for 2,000 years, and it achieves nothing but woeful thinking. Obsessing with the end of the world is a pointless exercise. It is written that 'no one knows the time of the apocalypse, except God. Not even the angels in heaven', so don't assume you *do* know something about it, because this has been a delusion for millions of people for centuries. Why waste your time thinking about something you have no control over? Just appreciate each new day in good health as a reward from the eons of life force, and honour the fact you have been granted consciousness. It is a phenomenal miracle with a plethora of underlying attributes that could allow you to achieve all manner of things. Many of the most successful people in life started out humbly, and yet believed in their own power. They never gave up, they never quit... they took charge of their own existences, and soldiered on through every minefield of problems. Think of problems like a puzzle in a computer game, a hurdle that needs to be crossed, or a puzzle that needs to be solved. Solve them... do not let them fester and develop in your own neurosis and escalate out of proportion. Accept the simple fact that, as a human being, you are here in the same way everybody else is, albeit in your own space and time zone, with a variety of cultural elements that will mould you to some extent. Don't let that moulding override your dream though, and don't surrender to what you have been instructed to as 'truth' per se - not even this letter - for 'truth' is as an ambiguous a term as anything can be, and yet many presume they've clinched the whole deal... When, in fact, they are potentially so far removed from what is actually 'the reality' that were they to glimpse the probable of the unseen, they'd alter their entire philosophy of life, and possibly be placed on state sponsored medication.

I knew a man who thought he was the most intelligent man in the pub once. He made sure he learnt a variety of things from books, and drank copious amounts of alcohol everyday, whilst speaking to the bar staff about all manner of philosophical, mythological, cultural, political, historical and literary instruction. However, I mentioned enlightenment once, and he told me I was 'talking shit'.

How wrong he was... At that precise moment, I knew that, however bright and knowledgeable a man might appear, he is not in possession of the facts of the higher truths. This is known to me, although I cannot prove it... but take it on trust. I am not lying. There is a prophecy from the bible: "They will be learned, but unable to know the truth". *Capiche*...

'Vertigo' plays on the stereo by U2, and it rocks. What an awesome track. It makes me want to fly a fighter jet on a mission to rescue humanity from the clutches of its own inadequacy.

Also know that the world is full of idiots… It's absolutely packed with them. Don't let them infect your equanimity. Banish their curse from your peace of mind. Just smile lovingly and hope they leave you alone… That is best.

Young Ashleigh, a work colleague, 18 years old, and fairly pretty has just come into the shop complaining about her life. Poor thing… so young, and so confused. What could I say to help her? Very little… I could say a thousand things as my mind revolved in her presence, but none of it would alter her own mentality. She is at the stage in life where you go from being top of the school of innocence, to bottom of the rung in the prison. I will be there for her where I can, of course. I am there for all those who need an ear to talk to. We're all trapped on this cosmic testicle in vast space… We need to get along, or we're done for…

Housed in the unit I am now in… my mind wonders… what will life's crusade grant me in this one man's quest for comprehension? What are my gifts? What are my flaws? How can I accentuate the positive and remove the negative? Surely they are both necessary energies, in order to create universal atomic balance? What must I do, in order to be liberated from the matrix? I cannot unplug my connection to society, or I would be at a loss. Although society is scared of me at times, I am not going to harm them. I wish them all the best. Go on fellows! Live long and prosper. Spock it to the max people. Spock it real good.

I digress... I shimmer and I quiver, and I await the passing of society's calibration of time so that I might leave this place of work, and return to my cell, to commune with my family. They don't particularly like me living there... but what can I do on my own? Half the world wants me dead it seems... I have experienced death threats from the phantoms for a decade. They're pretty useless assassins, I have to say. I'm still here, smiling, all *tickety boo* – waiting for the ancients of Moo-moo to rise again and explain exactly what it was they thought they were up to. But no... the ancients of Moo-moo (who were 'justified', as the legend would have us believe), are a curious breed, who shone universally for a second back in the 90s, and then fizzled back into the shadows of a multidimensional civilization that wondered who on earth they were, and what on earth they were going on about. It was all rather wonderful at the time, and apparently, one of their most treasured members drove an ice-cream van, which is a perfectly acceptable occupation.

The silence of the town corridors now teems with malevolence. How much of what the spirits tell me is true? What is the ideology in power really seeking to create in their running of the prison? Does Tone know what he's actually doing? Does anyone? Do I? Hello? Who are you? What are the dickens do you think you're doing?

Anyway... as I was saying... confusion is rife, and if you're not confused, you must be deluded. Complexity is everywhere, in every oscillation of the winds, in every thought in the brain, in every circuit switching on and off, in every illuminated pixel on the world-wide-web, in every quantum rotation of the nuts and bolts of this mammoth experience we call 'life'. To understand all that, is basically impossible... so don't give me this rubbish that you 'know the truth', because if you can't answer the two questions I will ask you at that given statement, I'll know you're a deluded person like everyone else. If you *did* know the answers to the two questions, and you hadn't already been informed; then, you probably wouldn't be claiming to know the truth in the first place, and therefore, I wouldn't ask the questions. What a cosy little paradox for you to savour for a moment.

I'll let you think about that one for seven seconds:

1... 2... 3... 4... 5... 6... 7...

Nice... Hope you enjoyed it. I certainly did.

Now... onto matters of utmost pressing concern. Hip-hop is celebrated by all manner of heathens

LOVE IN THE PRISON OF PSYCHOSIS

as a calling for truth. This is absurd. The majority of the culture revolves around sinister gun toting, horrendous methodology, and an unhealthy obsession with one's vanity, boasting and offensive / misogynistic lyrics. Let me show you why I don't respect Eminem as much as millions of his fans do. I will now freestyle rap for a small duration of time, without putting much effort into the poem I devise, just to illustrate how easy it is to create such words:

Yes, I'm like a terminator,
Just another annihilator,
Seeing the constraints of a system,
That might want to decimate all of yer.
Free flowing through the mindscape,
Caught in a heathen gate,
Reaping up the weeping,
Of the rendezvous that amalgamates,
Into a new form,
You're born into a higher storm,
Lapping at the juncture,
Of a function causing metaphors.
You're lost in an absolute,
Seeking to compute the loot,
That your father has acquired,
As a necessary input.
Into the system that derided you,
A rank of screaming platitudes,
A paradigm is such a crime,
When faced with hating attitudes.
But you think you know the benefit,
Of being born on top of it,

Nick Clark

A host of dying children,
And I'm still joyous in my element.
I don't want to see this torture now,
I think you thought I fought with clowns,
But I was sinking with the drinking,
Of liberated holy crowns.
And now I'm on the rebound,
Caught in the sight and sound.
Manifesting infestation,
Of an overriding compound.
That suggests to the west,
In their occidental splendour,
That their crimes of complaints,
Is anathema to remember.
And the society of sobriety,
That judges man eternally,
Is but another crutch to swing on,
In the face of apocalyptic tyranny,
And the ways that you appraise,
Unto the holy society,
Is but a method of control,
In these dark days of piety.
And the phase of the ways,
That coalesce unto the grave,
Is but illusion as intrusion,
In a silly sense of hazy days.
But the lyrics that pump your brain,
Are ridiculed by higher plains,
Talking about killing doesn't
Impress the kings, because you're vain.
And for a time we let it linger,
This trigger pulling finger,
Is placing flowers to the powers,

LOVE IN THE PRISON OF PSYCHOSIS

Because you've designed hysteria,
And the flow that will grow,
That is part of opposition,
Will deride all the lines,
Of decent supposition,
And you think you know it all,
By being involved in a brawl,
Where the fantasy of vanity,
Is leading to a fall.
And the notions of the oceans,
That like tsunami fill the motions,
A constant steaming of emotions,
And you still take out collateral,
But the mind of the time,
Is a higher form of practice,
Where the spirits of the ancients,
Appear just like an axis,
Of social misdemeanour,
A glorious czarina,
A slice of life, forgetting strife,
An enlightened ballerina.
Who will dance and sing,
'Forever' is what she brings,
A series of juries,
Could not quantify a sin,
When I was in the docks,
Because the world was on the rocks,
And the abominable ladies,
Thought of nothing sucking cocks.
And the way that we played with them,
A member of the brain playpen,
An holistic, futuristic,
Sense of theological zen,

Nick Clark

Believing in a higher cause,
A lion licking mighty paws,
Roaring against conforming,
When the order was a potent force.
So the methods they employ,
Simply to annoy,
Are totally lacking empathy,
In a world of silly ploys,
And the pain from the game,
That is your own name,
Causes you distress,
And again you've gone insane,
But I don't blame yer,
I just want to rearrange yer,
So that every facet of the tragic,
Is changed to entertain yer,
And the spiel I wield,
Without a sword or shield,
Is merely a momentary glimpse,
Into a society congealed.
By its own enforced neurosis.
They blame me for psychosis.
But what respect do you expect,
When they spread evil like osmosis,
And the plan you subscribe to,
Just another vibe school,
A system that's just dissed them,
And you're sitting like a proud fool.
Thinking you know what is what,
Just another robot,
Sitting computating,
As society feels the rot.
And the lame brain insane,

LOVE IN THE PRISON OF PSYCHOSIS

Mundane lower plain,
Seeks an answer to the questions,
That they can't even explain.
So the world spins on its axis,
And goes about its practice.
Thank heaven for faith in life,
Without it we'd be drastic.
And still after all these words,
I cannot align myself with murderous terms,
For the reeling in the feeling,
Is a deeper set of joyous verbs.
So we're taken to the ultimate,
A registered advertisement,
Of spies selling lies,
As I gaze into the firmament.
Golden light pulses through me,
You haven't even ruled me,
A mention of adventure,
And I'm now feeling supreme…

TIME : 29 minutes.

Most of that time was spent writing, as it all just peeled off the hippocampus, and therein, engineered an opening expanse of what it is to create rhyme in the hip-hop idiom. These rappers think they're so wise, yet with less than half an hour of free styling claptrap, I have written a series of lyrics that hasn't even begun to praise the gun. It's like the entire culture is an incestuous series of goats thinking they understand all things because under the influence of drugs, combined with a sinister mind, they can make a few words rhyme in this crime of the sublime. Where every little soldier in their ghetto reinforces you with a series of expletives as though it were poetic. What a sham and a mockery. A dirty, distant travesty. I'm still reciting lyrics even though I've changed my philosophy. So ignore the drudgery, of every zealous MC, when his ideology is simplicity, and his veneration of murdering is clear for all to see.

Haha...

WEDNESDAY 19th OCTOBER 2005

It's grey and raining... No surprise there then. A momentary tear in the clouds caused Earth's private star to pierce through hallowed light, but it has faded again to a drab climate of Stalinist slab misery. How this has an effect on the states of mind of the prisoners is debatable... but having once been allowed to escape the prison and visit Mauritius for a two-week sabbatical of intoxication, I long for such pleasant days again. I remember a waitress at the hotel we stayed at. So absolutely beautiful, yet coy. She takes up a few bits of ROM space in my thalamus. I wonder what she is doing now... To find such a lovely example of human flesh in such a distant Island is another of my own precious memories. A pathway only I have trodden, resulting in a unique state of mind, coated in personal recollections that only I have been privileged to view from my ephemeral scanning eyes.

LOVE IN THE PRISON OF PSYCHOSIS

Such memories I look to in order to deal with the moments I find a chore. Like Charlotte... One of my first loves. She was a blonde haired uber babe... How passionate we were, in our fleeting romance, and how potent her memory still is, lingering in my batch of recollections like a triumph of my narrative. I would love to see her again, but she is no doubt housed in another special zone, undertaking her daily routine in order to be considered socially viable. I hope she is doing well, and I hope she still thinks of me at times. She had a massive effect on my system of decisions. She was a vortex of beauty that whirled in and out the sphere of reference that is my personal reality. So, you see... The prison isn't always glum. Even under the tortuous presence of overriding thought control, it still bestows its charms betwixt the moments of solitude and despair. These are the points of your existence to cling to as a series of minor victories. A delightful and heavenly glance at what might have been should fates copious branches and rivulets of destiny have taken another route.

But now it's Danni who keeps me striving to exist, and bring about the blossoming of a heart formed from the miracle of creation. Were we not both so entrenched in the conventions of our own limitations and conditioning, we might have found ourselves entwined in a passion long ago. However, it was not to be... The fact I had had my mind thrown into the far reaches of outer space in a momentary divine manifestation long ago meant that I could no longer relate to fellow prisoners on a fundamental level. Her idea of 'truth' is still forming, but she is primed to embrace a great future, should the powers that guide her decision-making contain the necessary factors one requires to escape the prison. She has the best ticket a woman can possess to abscond from the lower echelon... incredible beauty. Most women in possession of this boon can utilise it to their advantage. I hope she does...

So now I linger in the void, derided by the locals at my pub for being too controversial and radical. They are afraid of so many topics of discourse, due to the problems of mind expansion they can never conceive. They retreat into their limited zones of reference so that they might not be seen for the timorous minds they are, and speak only of temporal, state authorised activities that comprise the prisons traditional notions of what is acceptable. Gambling is becoming a focal point for their social interaction. Such a foolish endeavour, but something to break the monotony of their daily routine. Talking of politics is another little aside from the terror that is their own deficiency, but such antiquated notions of mortal Governments bore me rigid, and serve merely as a series of humanoids playing a game of advanced chess. Where society is saturated in sound bites from leaders who primarily seize authority for their own personal egomania. Much of what they say has to speak to the masses, so that their overall oratories are abundant with simplistic concepts and civil matters of common sense. They do not embrace much in the way of cutting edge dynamic, visionary methodologies, but cling to the reactionary values of a society that championed a host of celebrities who now seem naïve in retrospect. I'm sure the same will happen for our generation, when our children's children are in control, and we will watch with grey-headed disgust as a whole phalanx of new ideas and media appal us in our geriatric slump. We will, no doubt, enjoy the programs we enjoy now, like the elderly still watch the repeats of programs that remind them of their days of glory. We will, no doubt, still be moaning about governments, tax, standards, behaviour of the youth, foreign policy, social pariahs, and the shocking stories of amazement that bombard our senses on the news. And so society continues in it's moulding, in it's obsession with the information it is given, and guided by hidden minds to a controlled and peaceful, productive system that contains millions of souls all quibbling about the same old things.

On the off chance that something radical was to present itself en masse to the inmates, no doubt its potential would far outweigh its ultimate practical implications, and the dismay following the triumph of hope will circulate again, and again, and again. Until one day, unless we have destroyed each other through utter madness, we might align our souls with the cosmic, and dwell in enlightened states of advanced thinking.

Lest we not forget the horrors of the 20th Century, the bloodiest of all, and the millions who died at the hands of extremism. Let us promote peace as the only course of action available in a world of weapons of mass destruction, and let us develop technology and learning to a state that we cannot even perhaps foresee at this juncture. My granny lived until 102. No way could she have known the changes in society that took place during the span of her years. The car, the computer, the plane, the genetic map, the power sources, the discoveries, the medicines, the literature, the music, the cinema, the television, the philosophies... It, no doubt, all immersed itself into her brain during her tonne and double years in the prison as a gradual development, but to leap from when she was a baby, to when she departed – the change was immense. Why should it not be the same for us? Who says someone with enough genius could not invent a *replicator*, or a quantum computer, or, even, a whole virtual universe of our own design, where we can escape by being constantly connected to a mammoth electronic housing system that grants us superhuman powers in a virtual domain. Think the Internet is advanced? It's only been around ten years or so for most people... What might it be like in 50, or 500 years time?

Everyone thinks they're right... And even if they don't claim to think they're right. They think they're right claiming to not think they're right... Another seminal paradox.

LOVE IN THE PRISON OF PSYCHOSIS

So I subdue my lucid brain for the pallid full moon beaming its fulgent ivory glare amid the molecules of the clouds as I drink a lager and tug on a cigarette, and fully realise the cosmic, as Jim Morrison sings 'Riders on the storm' from my terminus. The moment is different to all others, as are all moments... Even though I complain of routine, every 1 millionth of a cycle of the Caesium atom alone is a varied point in time, and, being the culmination of a number of intelligent biological properties, I can catalogue this moment in my one actual presence as a pretty swell sojourn into the meaning of a being. Titles for this book flicker through my mind's eye as I seek to select the precise name that will encapsulate all that I have scribed, and the latest is 'Kurtz E'. I feel like Colonel Kurtz now... I will never forget the line from 'Apocalypse now': "You can firebomb a whole village of Vietnamese, but you can't write 'fuck' on a bomb, because it's obscene".
I find that hugely powerful. One of the few quotes from cinema I recall. Colonel Kurtz is a legendary cinematic figure... An absolute genius. The darkness of his world is phenomenal, and the complete disregard for human life and disrespect for his nation is dripping in frightful malevolence. He is a monster of psychology, the deep jungle seemingly representing the depth of his mental anguish. I consider him phenomenal as a character, but seemingly opposite to me. I like the light, and the light is where I try to dwell.

Time: 10:25pm – Thursday 20th October 2005

Now I know why there is a hell... The subjects of many a dominion are so coated in dark thought, that should their nefarious thought process be allowed to control the system, the world would descend into chaos quicker than a sparkler lit by a blow torch on a hot day in Marrakesh. My God... how I have seen into the decadent process of logic the heathens provide unto their modus operandi, when they spin nothing but a pitiful horror of class ideology masquerading as power in the field of the horrific. No way am I planning on having children at this point in time... No way am I planning to bring another soul into this prison of horror. I hear, and I see, and I know just how despicable the methods are by which these people subconsciously construct their ideas. They're heathens... washed up, sickening, third world, lower class scum suckers clinging to the banks of a tortured river of warped emotion, whose faces should be tattooed with tiger stripes. They are the renegade elite of the Satanic incarnate. They think of rape of the innocent. I tell you, I would cut the throat of any man who dared harm one hair on the head of my angelic sister.

I walked back from the pub tonight feeling typically powerful, but with plenty of detractors... However, I felt I could wipe out a whole village in one night if they wronged me at the level I see in my psychosis. If one element of threat were deposited within my angelic sister's experience of existence, I would wage war with nations. I would gladly nuke a whole continent, knowing that the world was a malevolent species of pure sable hearts of ruin. Such thinking is anathema to my vision, and God's alike... and in so doing; I will create unending hellfire for all those opposed to the sanctified wonder of the awesome innocent. I will cut their throats, and I will throw away their heads, and urinate in their mouths for the kind of horror they espouse as wisdom. Their names will be removed for eternity from the book of life, and I will decimate their souls for eternity as the anarchic holocaust of retribution annihilates the very essence of all their sorry arse existences ever stood for... I will stab their eyes, and feed off their mother's blood, and stain their heritage for millennia, just because I know that their kind will not be tolerated in the palace of the almighty.

They talked of planets at the pub last night, while I was undergoing my latest trip into the latest void of despair due to the ominous voices... Their minds have gone interstellar, and inmate Rod tried to class the circumstances as a matter of Saturn. I disagreed, and spoke of the planet Lucy...
"It's not Saturn... It's Lucy... but it's too far away, too compact and it's made of solid diamond".
This seemed to make sense at the time... But inmate John looked at me with complete bewilderment. He never understands me... but then, I call him Mr. Cube secretly, because he's so square, he's three-dimensional. He's never once smoked a joint, and thus cannot comprehend the sensations of the illuminated soul. (I believe the soul is the energy of the nervous system). He has

never stepped outside of worldly trappings, and shone like an angel in the rapture of the awesome. I believe anyone who has never smoked a joint is a coward, and conjecture with regard to drugs is their Achilles heel. I know it is fear and ignorance that prevents some people from taking that leap into the great beyond... because it's the same reason I've never done crack or heroin... Fear, fear is not my ally. Fear is the path to the dark side, but with the faith in my revelation of the divinity, I can handle most of the virulent spectres emanations that plague my senses. Alert, lucid, honed... I await the next crisis of psychology with relish, for although I may die a tortured soul, I'll know for eternity that I entered the apotheosis of the chosen, and therein, I embrace all the devil might throw at me, because I'm light immaculate.

I ask that you don't judge me for the statements I have made in this tirade of the mind unleashed... because I am not alone in suffering these *malisons* of psychology. I repent for the evil in the last two pages, but simply sought to illustrate how much disdain I have for the thoughts of the wicked. I used to attend pottery classes for the mentally ill, and have met many people who suffer from a variety of conditions. They are scared and frightened people in the main, and I ask that if you take one thing away from this, it is that you do not slander those who have suffered from a mental health problem. 1 in 4 people will suffer from a psychological condition at some point in their lives, and the stigma it generates in society is deeply unacceptable. You could call all manner of people 'mentally ill' depending upon your belief system. The very fact our sensitive beings are so caught in a vortex of chemicals warping our reality is an aspect of creation and being human. Besides, you've never met a more interesting chap than 'Ray', who attends the pottery class... He's the fourth person I've met who thinks he's Jesus.

Another of the messiahs I've met did a talk for 'Voice Hearers'. He told us the funniest story I've ever heard. During one episode, he believed he was Christ returned and he ran to a church to be crucified. Prior to entering the sanctified chambers, he realised he needed to have 'the last supper', so he ran to McDonalds and purchased a chicken and egg McMuffin.

He then entered the church, and ran up to the priest.

"Who are you?" exclaimed the priest.

"I thought you'd recognise me..." he said.

So now I bring this letter to a close, and ask that you remember my creation at least with some moderate respect, for it was carved in words from an enlightened mind that seeks to illuminate you in subtle ways.

May you take from this series of terms and words (the variables by which I have designed this new program) a new thought process – one that might take you higher into liberty, but not the freedom of a form that is immorality. I don't expect you to be a saint... but at least show restraint, when faced with a situation that could result in a whole lifetime of recollection and guilt. May these gilded pages leave you pleased, even though the prison can seem so inhospitable and wretched at times, with its vicious entities and unfair aspects. You do not become totally suppressed by the platitudes and warped methods of the wicked, but find solace in the fact that there will one day be a great paradise.

Don't let the walls cave in on you... We can't live on without you.

Sincerely,

Inmate Nick Clark...
Mind expansion department

Solution...

The L shaped lump of cold steel precision engineering lay in my lap as I considered my options. The handgun was the first real one I'd ever been in possession of, and buying it moments ago from a devil in the pub was the ticket through the doorway to 'bad fate', should I not have been wise.

LOVE IN THE PRISON OF PSYCHOSIS

I never conceived of this taking place at university. I always intended to be a decent middle class son who would work hard, get average grades, a job, a beautiful wife, two point four sprogs, and a life of family values in Tory heartland... But a history of emotional pain required some kind of superior remedy than the Lustral and Abilify I was now on due to years of narcotic experimentation and crass mistakes.

Where does one begin to explain the ingredients that created my present state of mind? My personal histories wealth of various good and bad moments still clung to my adult mind over half a decade since the real problems had taken place. Ever since then, I guess I had been so drugged on mind control sedatives, that I hadn't appreciated how much the problems had affected me. Now I was awake again... Now I could see how much a few people, some of them supposedly 'friends', can have an effect on one's life in retrospect. Dominic was the worst offender, and the first bullet was for him. God... How I loathed that dyslexic, sex mad cretin who had shagged my girl. I had puked for a week after realising their little plan to try and dishonour me. Since then... Five years... I hadn't gone out with a girl again. Too damn emotionally horrific. I'm not going to gamble my sanity on the disgusting evils a modern corrupted bitch in a sex mad universe can manifest. Fuck that. I have serenity and peace of mind operating solo... But vengeance is still required, if only to regain my self respect.

So there I sat, in my silver Volkswagen golf, weapon in my hand, checking the trigger, clip, barrel, and bolt action for impurities, admiring its heartless and meticulousness design. I was not fooled though... Black clouds of cerebral anger enveloped my brain in darkness as I imagined taking out the target professionally – using the basic military training I had at private school, and a morsel of blind hatred.

I had contemplated the action for months... If I left him to be free in this world, the only justice he'd face would be perhaps a remorseful occasional sense of guilt – but he was psychotic. Guilt wasn't an option. He would, no doubt, have seen himself as a legend for his crime against me, and I had not even wronged him once. He thought I was evil, because I was often gravely serious and moody. What he failed to realise was that I was serious because I was in so much emotional pain – nothing to do with evil. Dominic was a cocaine dealer on the side for goodness sake, and once shoved a woman naked in a bush after he'd finished taking her from behind in a pub car park (which he boasted about). He thought *me* evil? Good grief... the ignorant prick was Satan himself, and my ex had fucked him with pleasure for reasons I would never know.
So... I could allow the psychotic to live free, knowing how much pain and rage he'd caused me, or I could unleash my own brand of personal judgement, and send the demonic cretin back to

LOVE IN THE PRISON OF PSYCHOSIS

Hades, where his sorry soul belonged. The choice now was heading in only one direction, and the addiction to the idea of how much pleasure I'd glean from seeing terror in his eyes, and then silencing the devil for good was burgeoning in my soul like a drug. Hell... Moses had even killed a man, and according to the scriptures, he was already in heaven. Conclusion... One kill isn't so bad... especially if it's pure scum like Dominic. God would no doubt be pleased with me for cleaning the social filth under the rug... After all... Come the Apocalypse... A whole load of scum we're heading down to the pit, and I didn't plan on joining them – however much carnal and immoral fun they had on this plain of reality. If you learn one thing from me... It's that a bit of casual sex while betraying one who depends on you isn't worth an eternity burning in excruciating sulphur...

I slid my fingers along the outside of the barrel and smiled. It was a quality gun. I'd gone to town spending on it, as I thought I should look the part. I didn't want an old fashioned piece with a six bullet rotary chamber like in the cowboy films. That design was old hat. I wanted a slick modern shooter, and, what's more, I'd done what all the best assassins did – added a silencer into the bargain. Silencers were, in my idea of a 'hit', essential. These Hollywood films with cops and felons running amok and firing loud weaponry randomly were so crass it seemed. So utterly anarchic and sloppy, like big kids playing cops and robbers for real amid crowded urban areas, and to hell with how much fear they created in the innocent bystanders as the slugs flew. To me, the professional killer always used a silencer, and didn't run about shouting, but used stealth and quick thinking as two major forms of protection. I would take out Dominic in silence – the pleasure would be mine – it would be 'my event', not to be shared quickly in chaos with his cohorts. It would be like a prayer answered, with me playing my own guardian angel – and seeing the horror in his drug-upped eyes would engrave my memory banks for good, a dark gem amid the treasure trove of my personal memories. Something to savour for the rest of time... Redemption from his historical presence in my existence, for his very life was like a cancer in my universe.

Did I think about the morality of my intended action? Of course I did. I studied theology at university, and it was thanks to immersing myself in the horrors of the Old Testament, and the blinding divine genocide of the prophecies which suggested to me that one little biddy hit wouldn't see me damned should I repented afterward. The Torah even celebrates some of their greatest warriors and war kings. David killing Goliath, for instance, or the mass slaughtering Samson. Well, I was David in the 21st Century, and Big Dom was going to feel the wrath of my creator, seeing as he was a Godless heathen. This titular king didn't use a sling though, he brandished high tech apparatus.

LOVE IN THE PRISON OF PSYCHOSIS

I sat and watched the outside scenery... I was wearing my fleece hoodie, and combat trousers as I licked my lips and considered the ramifications of the act. I would be technically committing a secular crime, but my religion wasn't the same as the rulers of the nation, and under a number of foreign religions, I would no doubt be absolved. Honour killings in Asia, killing of adulterers in Judaism and Islam, crimes of passion in occidental law, West Indian notions of tribal honour – they all had a basis in primal justification. What is more, the people who made laws in the West thought nothing of killing thousands of innocents in foreign countries with their missiles and advanced weapons of war, so one little kill that actually mattered should, in truth, go unnoticed. I stretched my shoulders, and felt my muscles tighten all over my torso. I was fit, I was agile, I was calm enough to dispense a cold bullet into a fool's head... and even if I were caught, I'd languish in jail with that bemused smile of satisfaction, given that I could officially claim insanity due to my schizophrenia, and get reprieve.

Gently pulling the stick into reverse, I drove away from the scummy area where I'd been tipped off about a small arms' dealer, and made my way back home, in order to prepare the mission.

I allowed my mp3 player to emit my selection of favourite tunes from my in car stereo with typical pleasure. Every song I had spent hours uploading into the miniature device was a song I loved. Thank the Lord for that splendid invention. If only I'd studied something useful like electronics, I might be a more successful man by now. 'Vertigo' by U2 punished the rear sub woofers as I negotiated the traffic ahead of me, and I smiled at the knowledge that such rock and roll heaven could be designed in a world so often dismayingly ugly. Like Dominic. Ugly. As though he proved evolution was real, and you could actually see the big nostrils, goofy lips, and thug jawbone of the primate hidden thousands of years beneath his stupid visage. Quite what Karen had seen in that imbecile was beyond me, other than perhaps a massive penis (he was known to be packing some serious length). This says more to me about the true nature of Karen's quality of femininity than it does about Dominic, to be fair. I despised the man... I despised Karen to some extent too, but I knew that I had loved her passionately once, whereas Dominic had always been a cretin. He'd driven home to a friend's house once after about six pints, and crashed his car, nearly killing a mutual acquaintance of ours. But nooo... I was the 'evil' one for being sensible and focused, and in pain. I didn't act like a wild fool, whose philosophy of excessive hedonism at any risk was the holy grail of life's meaning, and all detractors from such a juvenile tenet were the enemy. Prick. If anyone I'd ever known deserved rough justice, it was that swine. What's even more amusing... or worrying, depending on your point of view is the number of good-looking women he got. I guess it really is about cock size then, because they certainly weren't dating him for his brains, looks or money. He was in possession of none of the aforementioned. He laughed like a crazed hyena while so often chronically intoxicated, and managed to score with all manner of blonde bimbos. Confidence in egomania as aphrodisiac, but founded on nothing worth celebrating other than... er... a big dick. He flunked his exams at a private school, (which takes some doing), and then had to re-sit the third year of University, because he flunked that too, coming away with a 2:2 in Sports science.

I.e. He got a C in P.E after four years of training – and it wasn't like he was unfit – the amount of sex he got.

I drove back to my house, and settled the car onto the tarmac drive in the small town, where I wallowed in the shadows of my own personal pain. I would give about a couple of hours of my time planning the hit, and then I'd be out to the local restaurant to meet decent people, seeking an enlightening chat.

It just goes to show how insignificant the target was, due to the fact that searching his full name on Google came up with one hit, and it was a miss-hit at that. I could phone his father and ask where he was staying now, as I still had his family number (never get rid of information – you never know when it might be important), but to do so out of the blue would appear strange, as his father knew of the sin. No... I would have to go a slightly longer way around the houses in order to conceal my tracks, but my freedom depended on it. Besides... it was more fun trying to do everything perfectly right, when you knew what you were doing was so wrong.

Now... who would have his address? Who would have his number? I'd spoken to my friend John about him on the phone recently, idly inquiring as to his whereabouts. This was nothing out of the ordinary however, as I often talked to John about him, because there was a delightful reciprocated disgust for every element of his soul. It wasn't like I was one to talk about people behind their back either, but when you've been wronged by Satan with such magnitude, one believes they have a right to say something – anything – in order to unload some of the baggage, and possibly find a cure to the methods of the scum. Apparently, his best friend had been killed in a car accident a while ago, which, I hate to say, brought me no end of quiet satisfaction. Not for the demise of the friend... Poor chap... But the fact that it was Dom's best friend... His closest and most trusted ally... Deceased. Perhaps that was enough in the cosmic karma side of things. Perhaps having one's prime companion destroyed purely by chance *was* the justice I was seeking, but it wasn't enough for me. I hadn't suffered for years of emotional pain at seeing the pure ugliness of people through no fault of my own for such a conclusion by proxy. I demanded a taste of the action right in his face, to witness his last vision after 30 years of images. Me – firing a bullet into his forehead at point blank range with a contented smile. It would be poetry. I would be like an angel, glowing in the love of God's vitriolic assassins, dispensing rectitude of the unfairly wronged with a bullet called 'suck on this, punk'. (And he had been a punk in his teens; such was his level of intellectual ability).

I entered the confines of my apartment, and went up to the office space in order to work a bit more on one of the personal projects I was doing. I was designing a few web sites in order to get back at Karen. I could never kill Karen, even after what she had done. Although the pain of her grotesque betrayal was a daily cause of much suffering half a decade on, a distant, but powerful part of me still loved her immensely. She was my first love, and my entire soul for a time had been in paradise, as I believed naively that you could trust a woman. She was beautiful, fun to be with, and so, so angelic to look upon, but therein lay the paradox – no way was she an angel. She was a titian china doll full of maggots. So, I was not going to terminate her... I was simply going to play mind games with her. I had set up a fake 'MI5' site, linked to the main MI5 site, which looked as though she was on their 'most wanted' list for being involved with drug dealers. I was careful to copy the exact format and layout of the official MI5 site and fonts, including spending hours in

Photoshop designing the correct buttons, imagery, and touching up photos. When it was ready, all I would do would be to send her a link from an anonymous hotmail account, saying 'thought you'd better know about this'. She'd then link to it, and, if the ruse worked, spend her life looking over her shoulder. Even if it didn't work, the sheer pleasure in designing such a fun little game for me to dispense subtle revenge was a thrill nonetheless. I had photos of her, which I'd taken when stoned, wandering about in the garden. These looked ideal as 'photos taken from a spy camera'. Removing the colours, the black and white effect added to the illusion, which would have been generated after being brought up on a diet of modern spy thrillers. As I idly touched up the images and graphics, I allowed my mind to wonder how I might find out Dom's current address without leaving a trace. I decided that I'd need the help of an ex army friend, who now made his money hacking sites. He could get information on anyone, and he could also be trusted, seeing as if he was caught for some of the things he was doing, he'd be going away for a long time. £100 would be a lovely sum to pay for such delicious information, and a nice little earner for ten minutes work on his part. I would have to visit him tomorrow though, as I didn't want to leave a trace neither electronically nor telephonically.

So, that was that. I spent a while implementing my strategy, and then walked up to the restaurant to see what random selection of locals might be there to commune with. I knew they didn't respect me much. After all, I was hearing voices, and thought for myself. People around these parts didn't like that much. Any thought that you might unfurl into their ears that wasn't recognised as being 'official state policy' would be met with concern and mistrust. What they failed to appreciate however, was that I'd been to states of mind so high, so utterly divine, that most people simply reminded me of silly characters from a variety of British sitcoms, or cartoons in caricature. If they didn't come across that way, then they would be nefarious individuals I wouldn't give the time of day to. I can see where Peter Kay, Ricky Gervais, Ben Elton et al got many of their ideas from the more I immersed myself with mortals. Imperfection of human psychology was staggeringly prevalent. The amount of times I'd been slandered or falsely accused or disliked, purely on foundations that didn't stand up to scrutiny. Politics, religion, literature, the arts, philosophy, science, 'meaning of life', music, phenomenology... No... Most local people's ideas on these subjects were staggeringly limited, and I was the one taunted with a sceptical eye. "He knows too much" I would sometimes hear, and be socially lambasted and loathed. The phone hadn't rung for me once from a 'friend' in weeks, and my only crime had been to speak my mind. You'd think a friend would respect someone who tried to tell them the truth, but no. No one likes a 'know all wanker'...as I was often accused of being in the street. No way was I a 'know all', but in comparison to the seemingly total lack of quality data most minds seemed to be in possession of, I could understand where they got their small-minded opinion from. I was, in actual fact, deeply ignorant compared to the great minds that hid themselves away from the streets, earning proper money in plush buildings. However, a mere lamp amid a network of fireflies appears like a God when the sun isn't shining.

The usual assortment of regulars encompassed the rectangular bar at the restaurant, all in their expensive attire, not able to hide the less than attractive faces they were in possession of. It always saddened me, when ugly women would spend so much money on their hair, nails and expensive clothes. Didn't they understand? You can't make a dog into a Goddess, however much you spent on exterior dressage. However, a true beauty can have unkempt hair, sparse makeup, and be dressed in rags, and she'll still look like evidence of Helen of Troy reincarnated. A perfect piece of DNA, amid the chaff of thoughtless breeding. Rebecca was one of those girls. A stunning example of female beauty whose personality matched her physical perfection. When talking to her, the pain I felt on a daily basis would subside for a transient time, and her loving eyes and knowing giggle would radiate through my core. I never made a move on her, of course, because she was with another guy, and I respected her too much to think of having sex with her. It would be a sinful thought anyway, unless I was seeing her. Besides, that's one thing I hated about men…their ubiquitous, and utterly common obsession with sex, as though they thought they were 'cool', or 'knowing', or 'clever' to think of a beautiful woman as purely a piece of shag meat. Christ… These last five years had been so lonely, and increasingly surreal, as I tried to make sense of how non-believing society can live with itself, for all its perversion and biological freakiness. One of the regulars pointed out that a rather glamorous passing lady who I didn't recognise had a 'massive chest'.

"I wouldn't know," I said, "I look at a lady's face." This won me nothing but contempt and a description of 'arrogance', because I rarely fixate myself on the two lumps of absurdly shaped mounds swollen beneath a lady's jumper in polite society. These so called 'gentlemen' with their flash cash and successful lives are as morally decadent as any, so where the modern idea of 'class' comes into the picture, I do not know. Perhaps it is merely degrees of debauchery that ascertain whether or not a man's agenda is valid at a higher echelon or not. With a little creative imagination, I could be utterly vile, should I need to be. But unless I'd made millions by portraying it as 'art' in a film, I would be reprimanded. Not that I often thought vile thoughts. I merely mean it was not exactly hard to engineer them should I so wish, being in charge of my brain. No doubt they judge me harshly because I go into an expensive restaurant in a hoodie and combats, and not the utterly boring uniform of jeans and shirt. Man, I hate shirts… They look so dull… So lacking in originality or personality. They say nothing about a character to me other than he's a minion of 'the system of mediocrity' (or a fan of 'Magnum'). T-shirts, however, appeal to me much more, so I have my own designs printed up locally. I have one black T-shirt with 'DEUS EX' written on the back in gold Times New Roman. It may be a little vain, but by heck, it's like wearing a super hero's costume when out on the town. It sticks out subliminally a mile, and I feel like I'm such an individual, that I get feared and respected purely for applying two Latin words in gold to my shoulder blades. What's even more fun is that it fits nicely into the contemporary obsession with all things 'Illuminati', and although a little intellectually superior, it doesn't fail to impress. If only they knew I gave up Latin at the age of 13, and simply took the words from a computer game. Hehe…

Looking at the regulars, who are meant to be some of the heavy hitters from around the way still vaguely on the side of 'good', I begin to understand why some of Tony Blair's vision for the country failed to fall on good soil. He talked of a 'meritocracy', and seeing the lack of supersonic ideological genius in this place causes me to consider that part of the lack of Tony's success was: a) Because people can't live up to such high grade standards in the main due to chronic inability, and b) Those who did excel were generally envied by others. It was a rum do… and no mistake. So, I languished in my own thoughts while enjoying the effects of a pint of San Miguel, and studied the chattering classes with a distant eye, wondering as to the nature of their true thoughts. I saw society like an absurdly complex network of memory traces, where people's vocal emissions and behaviour all amassed into individual lives, and presented each person with his own completely unique and isolated mindset. This vastly elaborate multi-time based sequence of varying realities somehow congealed and hung together in a completely random experience, and yet people never seemed to talk of this. No one seemed to like to discuss life at this level, and seek to express how he or she honestly felt about the sheer complexities of sentient existence. Many were so 'normal' in their approach, thinking themselves 'socially authentic', that it was like living in the Stepford Wives or something. Biological robots all smiling daily because they had a rubbish job, got regular sex, and believed they knew what was best politically. I'd often lyrically depth charge a tedious scenario by saying an abstruse or abstract line, in order to test their emotional waters, and simply be met with a look of confusion. Didn't these people use their brains? Was it all a numbers' game to them? Was crude thinking and moneymaking the very limited be-all and end-all to their bizarre lives? Who were they anyway? And what the hell did they think they were doing by labelling me, judging me, talking about me? Like I give a rodent's posterior as to what they think of me... It's not like they've ever spoken to me at length about anything. They're so full of their own small-minded crap and ill thought through opinions that I'm surprised they don't explode under the pressure, leaving the walls stained in puss, mucous and muscle, the same components as anyone else. (Although they'd have you think otherwise - coated in their witchcraft finery).

I decided to pull back on the animosity, as it wasn't helping my equanimity, and considered the two albums of electronic music I'd composed. I really wanted to do a gig, but I felt embarrassed in case people thought my music was terrible. Personally, I marvelled at how, in the modern world, even someone with only one music lesson at the age of 12 could write pretty cool music using brilliant and affordable technology. I never knew I even had it in me. I sometimes play the albums I've composed while writing, doing websites, editing, or orating about whatever in a cyber commune. I think it sounds superb, and it even moves me. It flashes between dark and light, the relentless driving rhythm carrying the astral melodies and muscular bass lines. I'd love to have the courage of my convictions to play the music at a club, and watch the people flock to hear the sounds of 'me'... But, Alas... Luck hasn't been my lady for many a rotation of the moon, so I settle into my solitude, only my swamp brain for company.

The night, as is typical, turned out to be one of non-event. A few polite smiles, restricted divulging of opinions, a couple of fearful comments laced with menace due to some unknown sociological programme instilled into the minds of the lesser. God... I get hated for 'maybe' being Catholic, when the only Catholic thing about me I know of is that I spent five years at a Catholic boarding school – something completely against my wishes. So... I get persecuted and hated in the streets simply for something I had no say in. That's great, isn't it? Five years of being locked inside a mansion full of young men, only to be released, and hated for having been indoctrinated at great expense by 'whoever'. Jeesh... Someone pass the populace a brain please... I think some of them need cognitive upgrades.

I allow my thoughts to spin as I listen to the music. I smile lovingly as I think of that romantic moment in the car with my gun. It's quality... What a carefully deliberate construction. I feel amour for my soul as Kate Melluah sings a cutting-edge lament, and enjoy the notion of removing an official twat from the overly sullied tapestry that is modern society. I often consider global annihilation when relaxing over an evening libation. There is so much bloody darkness and hatred in the world that I sometimes wonder how the world managed to pull back from the brink during the Cuban missile crisis all those years ago. My dad would tell me how his parents picked him up from school on that day, thinking the end was actually going to happen. The story always fills me with emotion, as I think of my father as a boy, and my lovely grandparents brought to such a level of international paranoia that they believed they were all going to be wiped out over a philosophical disagreement taken to Defcon 4. I can only thank both the Russians and the Americans, equally, for not going the distance, for I happen to quite appreciate the fact that my existence has taken place, and aside from the horror I face from other imbeciles, I can still enjoy a warm bath in a warm house, and listen to the beautiful music of the era in blissful meditation. My mind glows with golden light, and I relax into such a deep transcendence of introspection and peace that sometimes I feel so peaceful, my heart might literally stop. The peace my own company can afford me in such luxurious calmness is stronger than any other fool's notion of what I might or might not be. How dare people persecute without motive. And they call me arrogant? What a joke. I don't look down on fat people or ethnics. I'm a very nice person. I may have the cold rage of murderous desire for being sinned against, smashing against my arteries as my blood turns to livid ice, but that is purely personal – it's not based on indiscriminate reasons. One of my theories is that in the future, due to globalisation, wars won't be fought and enemies won't be made in the name of nation and border. I'm not saying I'm right, maybe they will, but due to nuclear arms proliferation and a long period of international peace, it seems to me that unless another Hitler figure arrives on the scene, then logically, the enemy is a person you actually know personally.

LOVE IN THE PRISON OF PSYCHOSIS

After all, what beef do I have against, say, the Japanese, or the Koreans, or the Germans, or the 'Patagonians', considering they've done me no harm in this epoch, and yet scurrilous little demons I have offered my hand of trust to have treated me so appallingly? No, no... I won't be supporting 'my fellow country men' in a future conflict having suffered such ill treatment. I'll simply be waging a one-man act of vengeance on the mentally corrupt piece of soul crappiness that thought they had a right to wrong me with impunity. I would also like to smash in the face of Dominic's ugly mother against a toilet bowel, for housing such an ungodly piece of human detritus in her scabby womb... but I'm too lovely. I've never hit a woman in my life. I just simply seek to illustrate the rage one can sense when schemed against by pernicious and dyslexic minds.

Walking back through the streets of the town, I decided that whilst doing my rounds on the morrow, I would also visit young Emperor Dean. He wasn't a real Emperor though. At least, I don't think he is, unless he has underground power the magnitude of which he hasn't fully divulged – but he's one of the few people I know who has a brain of sufficient quality, and can drink me into oblivion. Drink is his soul appeaser, and he requires lots of medication at the weekend. He doesn't just speak to you when you visit, he lectures and orates, and is one of the most entertaining people I've ever had the pleasure of meeting. I considered asking his advice about the hit, but realised that telling anyone about my mission might be folly, however 'trusted' you think they might be. No matter... I'll just visit for a mammoth drinking session, and be shouted at every now and then, and then pass out on the couch giggling.

The absurdly beautiful stars filled the heavenly panorama as I sauntered back to my little brick shell, and I mused on the day's events at my place of work. I had had a discussion with Elias when he tried to buy 'Anti Christ Superstar' by Marilyn Manson that his soul was probably going to end up in hell for following false prophets. I tried to explain that angry riffs of such magnitude, combined with shouting demonic lyrics down a microphone was simply not cricket, especially considering that trying to be utterly disgusting in order to generate huge amounts of personal wealth was perhaps the nadir of Capitalism. Yet the guy sold millions of copies, and Elias attempted to mention how he'd been through hell in the past because of something someone did to him. I tried to make him see sense, and that listening to Satan was not the ticket out of one's pains, but his mind was made up. So, I sold him the CD containing nothing but faeces as euphony, and felt a flurry of sorrow as Elias left, wondering what had happened to him to make him think a Satanist was a saviour. How chronic... How philosophically moribund. The poor little chap with the scummy flat cap would, no doubt, sit listening to that harmonic filth, and imagine doing all manner of unholy things to whoever it was that wronged him. I dread to think how he'd been wronged... Probably some kind of sordid perversion involving brutality by a half-breed high on smack in the pastoral valleys of Hampshire one wet weekend. That kind of thing is never in the holiday brochures, and there's a damn good reason for it. So, as I walked to the door to enjoy a Marlboro, I noticed that there was a trail of urine on the shop floor.

Now... Either someone's baby had been lackadaisical with their bladder muscle commandeering, or a young foe that despised my existence decided to micturate on the parquet planks in defiance of everything I stood for. Either way, I cleaned up the offending liquid and went outside, where I met Josh strolling by. Josh was a smiley character, and with good reason. He was always stoned. The poor chap had been working for a 12-hour shift as a security guard on his own at a disused local missile silo, and had spent the time smoking joints. I was glad that the defence of the realm was in such good hands, as he told me he was sharpening his ninja sword whilst getting high. I immediately thought of 'Apocalypse Now', and giggled a tad to myself at the absurdity of the situation. Still, I wondered, what 'if' he had been attacked? Surely the drugs would have made him less capable? Surely being one man, high, was no grounds for a defensive position in the event of a hostile strike? Still... The chances of a disused missile silo in Hampshire being attacked if they only had one man on duty must have been slim. That kind of thing didn't really happen much in

Hampshire – as far as I knew. Besides, 12 hours on one's own, in the dark and the cold – one would need to be high just to make the time worth living. I'd go spare with insanity if I had to put up with a situation like that. Some jobs are so terrible, that they should have narcotic vending machines in the staff room to make the experience more bearable. Perhaps they knew he was a little pothead, and they just turned a blind eye to his needs and placed him in 'minimal security' so he could amuse himself on cannabis thinking he was Jackie Chan. Who knows…

Arriving back at my apartment, I chatted to a bunch of morons on the Internet for a brief duration. I decided after my third pint of the evening that arguing with a BNP supporter who repeated the line: "I don't givva fuck. You a coon loving faggot" ten times in a row because I chose to mention that I appreciated the work of Morgan Freeman, that enough was enough, and I retired. One major problem I have with the Internet is that the people who use the chat rooms often seem to be so poorly educated that you'd think we have vast areas of this nation filled to the brim with knife wielding savages, who cut people's throats for pleasure as they spew the saliva of crazed hatred. Aside from Hull, I can't think where on earth they reside. Not to matter… I dented the pillow, and slipped off into a heady dream.

Dreams do my nut in. Mankind has experienced them for thousands of years, and yet after all this time, no one is really sure what on earth they're for. The power of a nightmare can be hugely horrific, and the beauty of a great dream can cause you to wake with dismay as you realise what you thought was actually happening was but a surreal alternate reality taking place somehow in your brain. It was a whole weird deal…

On waking, I busied myself with having a shower and preparing myself to face the day. Another day, another twenty-four hour period at the edge of time, with the wake of 4.5 billion years trailing behind as though it all somehow meant more than it might. I ate a bacon sandwich in defiance of Judaism and Islam, and drank tea, in support of the last vestiges of Mighty Blighty's once great Empire. I then trundled into town, still thinking about my mission.

Nothing in the interim occurred of any note, until half way through the afternoon, when the absurdly happy Emily came bouncing in the shop, pleased as punch to meet me. The weird thing about Emily is that she is black. This isn't a racist comment. This is just weird because I live in a town where there are only about five black people out of a population of over 10,000. She would flutter her eyelids at me, and talk enthusiastically, and even bring up sex in the conversation. I didn't really know how to play the situation, as she was absolutely charming, but I knew from past experience that women could be the cause of much emotional torment. Besides, she might have been a spy working for the 'hip hop' movement, and been sent to find out whatever she could about me. You couldn't trust anyone these days – partly thanks to the X-Files. So, I would see how it went, and try to turn the situation to my favour. Although, I didn't particularly want anything from her – so I was all in a flummox. She kept on at me, saying how wonderful I was, when all I could do was stare at her rather large two front teeth. She would be so ebullient at meeting me, saying I was 'real', and lavish me with praise, when all the while I was wondering if she wanted my body, and if she did – what the hell would I do? She was coming on stronger than an Irn Bru Tsunami, and the butterfly lashes kept on fluttering. I naughtily felt a moment's arousal, but felt that she, no doubt, had a gangsta hip hop protection racket thing going on, and I'd be pissing off MC Bling Thing if I made a move on this little ebony fairy.

I kept control, my mind going in all directions, those tomb stone ivories still gleaming from the epicentre of a canyon smile. Her eyes glowing with fondness, her insistence I come to London to meet her on the verge of obsession. I didn't know what to do... I just kept responding politely to every given utterance, and then, after a quick touch and kiss on the cheek, she was gone. And I wondered if I'd eventually upset her father, the Catholic High Priest of Nigeria, by accident. Such were the ways realities numerous exchanges have of leaving strange cultural residue in the subconscious. I would remember this meeting of black meets white with much optimism. As though

LOVE IN THE PRISON OF PSYCHOSIS

a love heart had been thrown into a game of chess.

Afterwards, I had to get change from the pub as the stunning wife of the local copper cleaned out the till of change by using a ten-pound note. Funnily enough, I noticed the image of Darwin on the back looked exactly like our local's regular drunkard. Incredible... So I entered the bar to get the change, and there she was... Celia... One of the top local babes. She looked so radiant and the picture of female beauty, that I had to take stock of my entire physical embodiment with a focus on the matter at hand, and not order a pint of lager in giddy amour in order to spend the rest of my shift chatting the awesome babe up. I knew she had a slight crush on me... Nothing major... but I could see it in her smile, and the eyes darting excitedly in my direction... Or maybe she just fancied all men. She certainly had the beauty, and she wasn't dating one of the trendiest looking blokes in town because of her omelette recipe. No way... She was in the top five of the town uber babes, and my knees became molten with desire. Bravely, I got out of there, but not before asking whether she was off to somewhere special that night.

"No where... Why?" she replied, with a flirting smile that could get her into the secret vaults of Mugabe's Government.

"Because you look absolutely amazing... Best thing I've seen all day," I said, and made a run for it before I got too heated with passion. (Dealing with customers when you have an erection is never wise).

So... That brief moment with the fairer sex came upon me like a shockwave of random passing in time. There was definitely desire in her gaze. But see? See how like a foolish phallus wielder, I had been suckered into her gender web of sex crazed zeal? If I even made a move on her, I'd be doing to the 'trendy guy' exactly what Dominic had done to me. No... Cold water on the nuggets time. I must not let my virulent emotions lead me into darkened corridors of a woman's wicked power... I must be strong, like Ulysses fighting the Sirens. I cannot be a hypocrite, or... or... or... I will have to take the gun back and ask for my money back – which wouldn't be a good idea, seeing as he owned a whole arsenal, and was a crack head with strong opinions on refunds living in a slum with nothing to lose.

Damn... How stupid can I get? Ok... So my whole deal with Dom was because he destroyed my innocence. I suppose that's the real gripe I have. I had believed in true love until that moment, and subsequently realised it all a perverse game involving nothing but lust and secret thoughts of infidelity all centred round the slamming of balls against a pair of sweaty buttocks. Well... Muscular contractions and spurting juices aside... the gravitational pull of a babe's authority when she seeks a stupid male to pleasure her goes without question, and my radar had a massive glowing G-spot pinging at two degrees north-north-west.

Later on, she actually comes into the shop. Jeesh… She's returning a film, and my arteries are suddenly like scarlet rapids. I look at her, my eyes glowing in affection. Each time she comes in I speak to her more, probing her for more glances of desire. Little does she know what she's getting to know. She fails to realise I'm an agony mind; ruptured through betrayal of most of those I loved and respected. Venom pulsates through my chest as I spend hours in isolation waging mental warfare with lesser minds upon the techno reticulum 'simply because I can'. She doesn't know I have a crossfire gaze, and plenty of targets. She's probably aware that her delicate charm is but a cloak of emotional sorcery by which she causes men to act like loonies, but in my vicinity I have soul force-field protection mechanisms and mind upgrades. What if I told her I had discovered the 'subsonictron' while watching an evening news program?

I quoted a 'rolling stones' lyric to her in my supercilious obsession with trying to say things to people laden with potency, rather than this all too common secular denial that there is nothing supernatural about existence. There is… I am the evidence of that… but it's all a mind and soul thing. It happens at a higher level of reality that cannot be perceived by the non-believing. This is actually a 100% proven fact in my personal existence… but try telling that to a scientist who's foolish enough to have made his mind up about life. She makes the same face at least five times in the conversation, the amusing look I often employ: a diagonalisation of the mouth to suggest mock fear. She does it splendidly, and I like her even more. I am fairly strong in her presence, but I know to overstep the line and seek to create something more than what is hovering between us in emotional stasis would be corrupt. I smile a serious smile, and Annie Lennox springs into my mind - 'don't mess with a missionary man'. Yeah, right... Like I'm tough...

Either way, I wonder what she thinks of me at that precise juncture in space and time. She's certainly friendly, but perhaps I am coming on a little self-assured. I don't know... Thing's haven't quite been the same since she floated in and said 'I'm glad your fucking wanker of a boss isn't in..." as he emerged from the kitchenette. It gave me the giggles, I confess, but the air of embarrassed tension that that had generated now lingers as a video shop miasma of improper conduct involving mature adults.

Ha ha! Mature adults... I can't take them seriously. Half the people around society are weird... Utterly weird. A woman who gives her vows before God to a man who depends on her is often prepared to destroy that bond of trust when a handsome charmer makes all the right moves. Like Satan toying with Eve in the marriage of Eden. Shame... If I could get through the rest of life without thinking about sex with another woman I'd have to be some kind of prophet... It's virtually impossible, or do we simply live in morally corrupted times? I sometimes look at porn, simply because of its abundance, and it gives me the giggles. Sure, it gets me turned on too, but the women look so bloody ridiculous, while arousing at the same time – quite a paradox. Sex is comedy.

She leaves, and I return to my seat to add to my archives of personal events. White sparkles of angelic light flash like magic out of the corner of my eye, and I wonder what the future has in store for me. Will I find another love that I might trust? Or will I be forever cursed with the embodiment of a self-confident twat who thinks he's worth a damn thing, and knows virtually nothing?

Christ... My mind spins onto thoughts of my situation, and I smile pleasantly at least with the confidence that the babe once blew me a kiss – Naughty, as it was. The pain of loss returns to my shell of a body, and I force my faith power to override the insurgency of anguish, keeping above the capitulation to self-destruct. I must keep moving... I must keep laughing... I mustn't let the filth in society's matrix of strange ideas vanquish my lustrous nervous system. Keep riding the higher dreams... keep pure, alone, stealth like, strong, fighting the desires. Like a panther seeking prey in the jungle, or, at least, a moggy seeking milk from the kitchen in a nice suburban family home.

I step outside for a lung crusher, so I can people watch. A kid moonwalks in the street, and an aged vamp gives me the curious eye. Strangers carry various things as they lug their bizarre and obviously necessary wares hither and thither. It's coming up to Xmas, and I think a badass thought. Just imagine terminating my target on that special day. Crikey... How evil am I thinking? Or is that the true price of vengeance, to design a poetic demise using such careful stratagem, that the sheer blast of horror in the lives of my enemy will resonate through their lineage for all time, a blemish of dishonour of such scale, that it would become historical.

Perhaps... Or perhaps it would have this avenging angel sent straight to hellfire and damnation for such pernicious skulduggery. Who am I to say? I am not the Lord... I only know that a psychotic who uses religion as his basis for motive is a powerful mind indeed, however much worldly notions of justice dispute their methods.

The massive rupture of my sanity occurred while at university. Considering it was a place of learning, I made more mistakes than could ever be imagined. I had never been the same since 1992, when David and myself had gone into supernova on our first LSD trip. Talk about opening the doors of perception... We blew up the portcullis of insight and soldiered through into heaven and hell. I'll never fathom how much that experience was a formative influence in my entire existence. Ever since, I was an electrified roller

LOVE IN THE PRISON OF PSYCHOSIS

ball of psychedelic thought emanations that pinballed through time forever, behaving like a damnable fool in the eyes of normal men... But when you've laughed in friendship to such an extent, while zooming through the divine realms, and thinking you actually have a role to play in the holy battle between good and evil, talking about pensions at a pub with mortal men doesn't quite have the same exhilaration. So, my madness is not really madness... What it really is... Is like sodium in water. One volatile state meeting an opposing catalyst. Of course... Both are pure and natural elements of the universe, but some partnerships just create nothing but bad energy, and some none but good. It would be nice to know though, that if I wasn't such a deluded, high minded walking disaster of a 'petrol in water' brain that I might ally myself with another damaged angel, and cling together in the Zion meadows, swiping at the snapping demons with laser sabres, and metallic electric wings.

I desire the perfect embrace... the fulsome connection of perfect love caught in eternal splendour. The moron that I am felt it once, ("monopoly and properly kissed"), and in my juvenile ignorance, I left that place of gilded perfection in pursuit of more notches on the bedpost. What a bloody fool I must have been. I could have luxuriated in innocence for all time perhaps, with a female sidekick of exceptional pulchritude by which to share all the masterful methods of correct living. But alas... I am destined to walk alone for seemingly an inevitable time with pain my crutch as I struggle to unravel the equations of the mind. The grey matter that does not shine such dull colours internally reverberates unceasing, as I cling to the rigs of the higher plateaus for all I'm worth, nothing but the torment of a catalogue of histories folly's to plague my being.

The alternative is suicide... Self-destruction... I am inoperable with this amount of agony in a meritocracy, so how can I fend for myself on a daily basis? But suicide is not an option... Too damn low... Too ungrateful for all the good days I've lived and loved, and the family that's protected me. I could just seize the day, and get in my car, and head for India in order to live in the heat and live rough, smoking the notorious herb all day, but I'm lacking in funds. A degree in theology is not enough to grant me access to high earning careers, and I'm not sure I could stand the absolute tedium of working in a cerebral battery chicken enclave selling boring guff. The ruin at the foundations of my soul temple have cracked to such an extent, that it's half subsided into the precipice... but a spirit is what defines a person's essence, and who knows what might arise from the ashes of misery should I endeavour to listen to the holiest word I know: "Continue".

A man hobbles past the window showing the traces of weathering as he strives to keep going. I wonder what his history is... his triumphs, his failures, the seemingly random nature by which his genesis was forged in the annals of time to allow him to bypass my vision right at this point in

LOVE IN THE PRISON OF PSYCHOSIS

chronology. Of course, like so many moments in the street, nothing is said... it's not really the English way... as though we're all too important to deign to talk to other human beings, in case we give away too many state secrets, or worse, discuss religion. He ambles on. His joints require oiling. His walking aid positing dismay into my heart, as I vicariously dread to live with his ailments. He is the shadow of time; the portent of a life in youth lived carelessly. I spy the cigarette in my hand, and consider my idiocy, but then, I know Christian fundamentalists who haven't got the brains they were born with... What is time when young if not revelled in, and pleasure taken as a boon? The only young man I know in my generation who lived 'as they would have you', and spent many years sober suffered from depression of such seriousness, that he really couldn't care less if he died, and had often contemplated suicide. Why? He hadn't even royally screwed up at the level I had... He'd got a scholarship to a leading British public school, got a good degree... and merely wallowed in the mire for years upon years of self imposed misery. Jeesh! At least while the world was thinking me a maddened fool, I was floating on cloud 9000 thinking I was a genius of a new way of thinking.
No justice... A man saves the world, and he's persecuted by many for such valour, and a timid character acts like a good boy, dwells in pure gloom, and is considered 'appropriately behaved'. Brilliant... I'm so impressed with adult methods.

As I write these confused words, the pulse of an awesome modern dance album pummels my eardrums. It's utterly fantastic, like joyous angels of hope celebrating dance evangelism in electro munificence. I even have a young man dancing in the shop, with two teenage girls quibbling as to whether I'm cool or not.

Am I 'cool'? I don't know... What is 'cool'? Once upon a time, it was 'cool' to like 'Bros'... Another time it was 'cool' to wear flares... A pair of trousers so utterly devoid of anything I might deem 'cool' whatsoever, that I even thought of not recognising my father as my father due to one photo from the 70s in which he sports the absurd clothes. So, obviously, 'cool' is a concept of no officially defined basis that transmogrifies with time depending on trends and fads... So... I may be cool today... but tomorrow, I may be uncool... and then I may be cool again... Who knows? I'm usually a similar kind of guy. I suppose it's just dependant on how eyes fluctuating on cutting edge frequencies perceive me as a gauge for their own metamorphosing tastes from a quasi spiritual abstract character study.

Whatever... I jig to the groove, and find most satisfaction in this excellent selection of euphonies. I punch the air, and conclude I am a modern work of bizarre reality, given that we're living in an age where anything is virtually possible...

Anyway... I shouldn't be raving while at work; I should be suppressed by horrendous ideas of what it is to act accordingly. So, I simply feel the nauseous weight of agony emerge back into my body, and after twenty seconds of that, feel so utterly uninspired, that I crank up the dance tunes again, and jig on out the door for a vili flattener.

I am out there in the cold, watching the same old site I've seen for over a year, but this time my legs are moving to the beat that lingers in my heart. I have images of clubbers dancing in a wild frenzy of positive hope... I accept this as a far better alternative to nuclear Armageddon and, although they are, no doubt, draped in maddened sinful behaviour, you've got to admit it's a better vibe than hatred and fear disguised as religion. Besides, Hymn's sung in church have all the emotive celebration of an antiquated and cosmic time in yore when they did actually sound hot off the press.

People seem to think Christianity is an 18th Century English piece of organ music involving pseudo Shakespearian doxologies. What utter reactionary and foolish nonsense. The spirit is alive in all those who believe in love depending on the technology and literary trends of the current epoch... and it now uses break-beat in some higher-minded sects. These forward thinking electronic dance geniuses have taken my soul on a futuristic trip into tachyon souls and laser amour. I groove in my chair, with the positive bass line bringing together people of all backgrounds to the universal sound of music. Julie Andrews would, no doubt, have been into rave music in the Swiss Alps in her time, if her nanny affection for jubilant youth accepted these pulsing chords with relish, and not associated them with some kind of neo-Nazi conspiracy, utilising rhythm and subliminal vocals as a subconscious manifesto.

Next day... and I'm back again... in pain and tedium... Christ, I've got to get some proper money together... I need to get the hell out of here. I need to regain my hope... It's seeped out my backside like a callow runaway, desperate for departure from the chronic mind that has caused it so many wounds. Come back little hope... I love you. I need you. I'm going spare without you... The dreary music I'm listening to isn't helping either... It's the sounds of morbidity and self-loathing. It's basically a talented manic-depressive who re-creates the ennui of his personal grief for thousands to indulge in on CD... Quick... Reroute harmonic emission system disc choice, and feel the groove.

I opt for John Lennon, and sit back to enjoy another period of time from the perspective of an icon.

I need to neutralise my mind... My desire to kill my primary target is, no doubt, being punished by the Lord... But how can I continue with this shit? I'm sick of it... Absolutely sick of it...

"Imagine" comes on... And I slump back into this apotheosis tune, knowing it is virtually pop gospel for millions of unified dreamers.

Decisions... options... Time to enact a plan... But I can't terminate the target on Xmas Day... I need longer to prepare. Perhaps I will wait for his birthday. But no... I need to know that I am on the ball now... I need to know I am worth something to someone else. What's the point in existence if I'm not? Shit... I'm just another piece in the mental jigsaw. A spot in the mosaic of reality. I'm sobbing and giggling internally every five minutes...

That's it! I am actually mad... I am deranged beyond all reason... and yet... I speak so much more sense than some. I can actually spin a handsome verb around a flirting adjective, and allow a promising sentence to emerge from the slumber of a complacent world.

A couple came into the shop the other night, and talked to me as I tried with all me being to register their attempts at communication as something more than embarrassing garbage. They then had a brief argument, which, I kid you not, went like this:

"That film was based on a true story you know."

"No it wasn't"

"Yes it was."

"No it wasn't. Don't be stupid."

"It bloody was, it said 'Based on a true story' at the beginning".

"Oh yeah, it did."

Not only that, but I picked up on at least five facts the male got utterly wrong, ceasing to correct him after the first two for fear of being branded a pompous pedant.

The line from 'a working class hero' reverberated around my skull.

"They hate you if you're clever, and despise a fool." That is so true... So true it makes me mad... So mad that I want to unleash my rage by removing my T-shirt, and stand in the middle of the road taking on moving vehicles. But I won't... That kind of behaviour is not socially the norm, and I might get injured. We are trapped in the legislation maze... and a lot of bubbling minds are drowning in worry... Being an adult is the pits frequently... It's all a suspicious plot to remove the funk and fly of an impassioned free spirit hell bent on glory hunting. I won't be party to the conspiracy... I must return to studying the inner thoughts of my deep consciousness, where I on occasion stumble upon a literary gem, and wield a stream of images unto the collective mindset.

Shit... I should never have studied 'The Apocalypse' while on drugs... bad move on my part. Dunce to King twelve. I scupper my life on a regular basis by desiring to reach deep into the vast recesses of higher purpose, and garner from this miraculous strange phenomenon the essence of all that is meaningful. Maybe it's a guitar riff, or a flower, or a girl's adoring eyes, or the birth of a baby, or the excitement of a loyal friend, or a sense of overwhelming peace, or a piece of important writing. Who's to say? There are an infinite number of personal realities to explore, should people be a little more forthcoming. My friend told me last night that we are the 'children of the light'... Perhaps we are, and the future will soon be given to us in order to make the decisions that guide a host of nations... We can choose a number of options by which our futures will be determined. We must seek to choose wisely, and probably not actually get high as kites and shag each other's girls... For the latent distrust, pain and rage that causes in a collection of individuals might one day reach boiling point... Nihilism formed through immorality – a horrendous fate for millions... Yet it is so hard to spend an entire life living perfectly. So hard indeed, and quite unrealistic. It was alright for Jesus, he was the son of God, so he knew he was onto a winner. What about all the other less-than-prestigious babies spawned of cacker DNA though? Hmm? Not quite so easy for them is it? Thoughtless bunch, those religionists.

Thus, I subscribe to the philosophy that pain is a necessary aspect of the living experience, whereby we learn the meaning of rules and codes so that we might survive and develop into wiser, more decent individuals. For the nefarious nature of the psychotic, and why he is deemed so universally iniquitous is that he is devoid of emotion and conscience, and thus poses a plethora of grave dangers to the more benevolent members of a society.

We were made imperfect, and therein lies the genesis of our own suffering. What a pisser. I loathe so many of my thoughts... I can't believe they're actually in my head. I allow them to enter due to the free flow of imagery caused via association, but every now and then, a concept of sheer pernicious wickedness will permeate into my gelatine mind, and I will be appalled at the horror of where that disgraceful synaptic projection has emerged from. I blot it out, and sink lower into a concern that I am corrupt beyond measure. I tend not to revel in the disgusting, and try to keep my head held high... But the agony lingers like a tumour of dissatisfaction. I find that to sit with a clear mind, a head devoid of any real thought other than following the sober and wordy stratagems of an intellectual system, is the only time I can feel peace of mind. This obsession with the expiration of Dominic's malignant soul is anathema to a society founded on regulation, and although I know it is an erroneous thought process, I cannot help but become fixated, and I suggest that this unhealthy cathexis of iniquity is due to improper decision making on my part in the first place. I knew Karen wasn't 'the one', and for all the candyfloss surges of delighted passion that we shared, I knew she hadn't made the grade for eternity. So, I conclude that due to my impatience in desiring a female mate during the folly of my teenage years, I am now suffering the karmic recompense for such indiscipline. Nevertheless... I'll keep moving... I'll keep moving...

Like Bruce Wayne searching for the mountain fortress of the 'League of Shadows', I walk through the freezing winter air, the ice symbolising my heart, looking for the insight into my essence that will trigger in me the necessary information I require achieving my destiny, and winning my peace of mind.

I go to see Emperor Dean, and he invites me into his small concrete box. We go through the same initial stages of the 'Dean experience', which is Dean being grouchy at the dog, because it is

LOVE IN THE PRISON OF PSYCHOSIS

hectic at my arrival, Dean being grouchy at the kid, because she's being excitable at my arrival, and Dean being angry with me, because I say something he deems utterly facile. As is traditional with the 'Dean experience', he then turns from a mode of utter disdain into one of total pleasantries, and offers me a beer, which I gratefully accept. His girl, Empress Summer of the Northern Tribes, tests me in her strange female ways, and like an eight ball oracle, I will be met with one of a few methods of retaliation to my comments. (Facile as they are). I never quite know what to say to Emperor Dean, as he has the mind of a genius, the haggard face of Colonel Kurtz, and the history of a legend.

Whenever we have our marathon drinking sessions, I impart about one sentence to fifty from him. Ratio – 1:50. That is not exaggerating either. When I do speak up, I am rightfully told to just let Dean get a word in. I think Dean's mind frequency, when vocalised due to intoxicant lubrication, is at such a high level of speed, acumen, and agility, at least in the first six pint stages, due to a history of dealing in a hard world of hard men doing hard things, that he has lost the plot in some ways. I come from a fluffy world of fluffy people doing fluffy things, and thus, whenever Emperor Dean, of erudition unsurpassed comparative to that of the rest of the local populace I have so far debated with at length unleashes, I rightfully shut-up and listen. Not only that, but were I to enrage his mighty heart, filled with wrath as it is at the best of times, I might suffer a serious kicking. For which I, of course, would be eternally grateful, because I would have had the shit kicked out of me by Emperor Dean, and not actually sent to the front or killed, and his mercy would linger in my heart like a rose petal on a barbed wire slinky.

The evening started with the typical bout of Emperor Dean playing loud, often frighteningly angry music as he knocked back glass after glass of the quick knicker dropper liquor, and orates to me about lyrics he finds meaningful. I accept his views, and appreciate the different ways minds are forged in a society filled with a million alternate moments in space and time that are now entwined at this absolute current juncture, seeking to commune at some level of rationale and insight. Of course, every time I utter something, it is usually met with a complete mocking farce, for he has led platoons of pub heroes to victory in foreign lands, and I have eaten Spicy Curry Pot Noodles on dope at university thinking I was being cultured. He stands with a general's hand in his inner jacket, clutching at his chest when he speaks at length on all matters of existence, the pointlessness of life, the depths of despair, the boredom of all things, and the occasional moment of laughter at some cynical comment from whoever may be contemplating suicide in his presence. I then seek to stand up for my beliefs in life being some kind of heavenly gift to treasure, and am vocally cannoned into silence due to such simple minded rhetoric. Any talk of a higher divinity is routinely met with absolute disgust, and even though I wield a halo, and sometimes sense

LOVE IN THE PRISON OF PSYCHOSIS

astral, angel wings protruding from my back when I am absolutely high, I realise that the entire existence of mine must be a delusion, and that anything that occurs in my mind or spirit is of no consequence whatsoever, and should be ignored due to it being 'not of reality'. When I seek to explain that 'reality' is an illusion envisaged via a biological computation system made mostly of water and definitely possesses latent abilities to make contact with supernatural forces, I am dismissed, of course, for 'talking shit'. Then, everyone sits down in a state of depression because I am made of pure energy, and no one wants to dance to happy music, but instead wishes to wallow in the mire of material inequality, and 20th Century notions of class injustice.

"Happiness is a brave sentence of honesty spoken to a stranger in random time," I might say, for instance, and be looked at by Emperor Dean, of course rightly, with a raised eyebrow and sneer of disapproval, due to it not being compatible with his ingrained series of philosophical precepts. For only Emperor Dean knows the truth, and I am but a prevaricating arse with stupid notions who should be silent at all times, unless telling Dean to 'carry on, I'm finding this story interesting'. I then drink myself further into oblivion until I can only see the lectures through a thin and diffracted light beam of half closed weary eyes, until I surrender into fatigue and drift off in a complete bamboozlement.

Next morning, everything is chipper again.

"Cheerio Dean!" I say, after a lovely cup of tea.

"Cheerio Nick. Same time soon, wot?" He says, and we leave on a jocund gag as I try, at the best level of all my reason, to fathom his methodology after living in quite an alternate universe to him for my entire life. Although I appreciate that Dean, with a touch of the Job about him, sees life as utterly pointless, I consider this so amusing, (even if it's correct), that I laugh all the way home, and think 'life can't be pointless... laughing is fantastic', and therein conclude that life is pointless laughing... and therefore, mad people are the closest to self actualisation.

Well... It makes sense to me...

So I arrive back at work with a hangover that could lose the Iraq War, and sit on the stool of bum remoulding severity due to its immense plastic rigidity for four long hours of solitude, listening to 80s albums, and realising that I need a serious discussion with David.

David, the ally I spoke of earlier, believes that the 80s, and I quote, 'should be deleted'.

I am appalled at this, as much of Annie Lennox and Mark Knopfler's work, to name but two acts among many, seem to be so superior in musical beauty than much of the 90s. (Which to me was like living in Nazi Germany without the violence and death). I also plan one day to sit David down on a rather plush beanbag, and make him listen to Dire Strait's 'Money for nothing' and 'Sultan's of swing' (probably while stoned), and compare it to the 'so called most important album ever' – Nirvana's 'Nevermind'.

LOVE IN THE PRISON OF PSYCHOSIS

Now, forgive me if what I'm about to say might be construed as rock and roll blasphemy, but these two Dire Strait's songs evoke in me more power, beauty, rock and roll glory and sheer talent than the dirgy, grungy, simple angst of the muddy Hippy in a woolly jumper from Silicon Valley's environs who produced the seminal album of guitar destroying pain. I mean... 'Come as you are', and 'smells like teen spirit' are cool tunes... Nothing life shatteringly transforming, though. As for the last 'hidden' song (track '13', I think it is), which blasts onto one's speakers long after the official last track has played... Well... I'm sorry... But it's like the sounds of hell, and quite how any half intelligent mind of even some personal well being can find favour in such a cacophony of harmonic dissonance is quite beyond me, and thus, I think half the white 20-30 something's of the modern era led stupid adolescent lives of egomaniacal delusion, and couldn't explain in intelligent detail anything of value other than 'it spoke to my heart, man'. (Ergo, that pumping morass of blood cells reverberates with the sound of a freak composing a lot of rubbish that did nothing but make the 90s all too often a backwater of insecurity, paranoia and emotional pain). It was in the dance world where the 90s really took off in my humble opinion and yet the Prodigy, probably the pioneers of the rave generation emersion into mainstream society, became darker than a coal moon, quoting neo-Nazi propaganda. Crikey! What the dickens is that all about? Am I completely out of touch? What the dickory-dock is going on in my generation? Are they really all Satanic bastards?

My theory is that the naughty little denizens of the national hood are beginning to see the darkness as light, and the light as dark. I know... I've seen it, and it smacks of naughty psychology. They wade through the cognitive depths of a dark rock tune embellished with anger in a world of plenty. I blame this partly on communication. We see more about the world we live in than 100 years ago, and more wickedness too is displayed on the screens. This festers and builds, and swirls within our craniums, it taunts our morality, and it plagues our senses. It displays the horrors of the Earth on prime time channels, and the comedy is so faux on occasion, it seems like a nefarious conspiracy to some. The obsession with perversion, sex, guns and violence bombarding our retinas on a daily basis is surely reflected in our souls and minds as it's like a gallery of temptation, an aquarium of tantalising fantasies.

Thus, in pursuit of the championed notion of 'pursuit of happiness', we leave a wake of emotional wreckage in our historie's course as we always think we need more. We must consume, and consume, and yet... As we forever feed the capitalist Empire that gave us such halcyon upbringings, many turn to internal rage as the dream we were sold in our adolescence fails to materialise en masse. We're allowed to revel in 'freedom' on occasional weekends throughout the year at festivals, but those festival's acts have all too commonly been polluted with degenerate and immoral musical groups, who, no doubt, do nothing but further cause the zeitgeist of a nation to flounder and collapse into emotional despair – masquerading as celebrating our pain. The antithesis to this is the dance scene, where ugliness is often prohibited, due to an obsession with vanity and 'intellectual' snobbery. The traditional bastions of classical music remain in stasis, and old school parties of music from the 50s to the 90s seem outdated, as the pursuit to be cutting edge on a weekly basis grinds at the national framework, causing a polarising into multifarious and strange new sounds found on the Internet – the electro Babel.

"I think you worry too much," came the voice from inside my head, as I punished the sable keyboard with all the venom of a man vocally wronged by a thousand strangers whilst skyrocketed out of my brain in... 1995, was it? Perhaps it was 1996? Something weird happened in 1997 too... and 1999... Which leaves 1998 floundering in an oasis of its own – but I have no idea what happened then. I suspect I was out of it.

(Jesus! There's a mother in the shop who has the voice of a man...)

Anyway... So whilst I was cruising through the mental part of the latter 90s, Lord only knows what happened to my faculty for reason. If only I could explain what might, or might not have occurred in that time frame. It was like a colossal head-trip into the psychotic realms of complete perhapsness. I laughed out loud in the bath last night as I found a diary from the year 1997. There were so many entries that were out of their mind. I thought I was an angel for at least the better part of a year, after I was placed in the Priory for over indulgence of that God-awful drug LSD. (Lethal Sense Decimator, as I call it). There is also a sentence written in bold after I had returned from Glastonbury festival one year. It simply reads, underlined:

"YOU ARE NOT THE GOLDEN LAMB"

Talk about weird. Although, if the truth be known I still to this day know what I was going on about. There is a lot of writing about God, and a revolution that might or might not have happened. It's hard to tell.

Advice: Never try to start a revolution surrounded by thousands of believers when high, because:

a) They might actually believe in you. Which means,

b) They might actually follow you. Which means,

c) They will expect results. Which means,

d) You better be pretty good at getting the job done. Which means,

e) It's not wise to be high. Unless…

f) They are all high too, and simply think you're beautiful for shouting 'Revolution!' while high as a kite, because you studied a bit of Marx at private school politics A-Level and think he was a boring git, and you could do much better, because, 'like, God actually spoke to you' once while you were on magic mushrooms in the local Off License.

LOVE IN THE PRISON OF PSYCHOSIS

However, if they are fairly intelligent themselves, and really think you're the man for the job... Then:

a) You really HAD better get results. Which means,

b) You really shouldn't be high at all. Because,

c) They won't be impressed when they say: 'So where is our food and shelter?' and you shout 'THE ALMIGHTY RA, GOD OF THE SUN, WILL FEED US WITH LIGHT FROM HIS AWESOMENESS'. Leading to them saying something along the lines of 'but Vitamin D is not rich enough in protein and sustenance to keep a homosapien fit and healthy for years on end'. To which you say, due to chronic intoxication, 'Oh, feck it... The revolution won't work anyway. I know nothing about running a stable economy, and I can't see how we're going to get past the global warming crisis without..."

And then you realise what you're about to say... And stop mid sentence, because the idea is so utterly frightening, potentially, and you might be wrong anyway, because you're a stupid theological student/artist who is very good at coming up with ideas for science fiction films, but doesn't have a clue as to the realities of ozone depletion testing among other things. So you remain taciturn and reticent having just had, at least, a thousand people follow you right into the heart of their opposing tribe of non-believers, and there you are, all these people looking at you, seeking guidance. And then, because you're high, the memory of 'The Life of Brian' pops into your head, where Brian shouts from the window "You are all individuals!" You can't believe this is actually happening, so piss yourself laughing, and then everyone is finally convinced you're madder than a lead hamper of glowing squirrels, and they walk off complaining that 'you're full of shit'. To which you become quite peeved seeing that you, at least, made it all the way through private school obtaining some good grades, even though you were asked to leave on the last day as they thought you might burn down the school or something, and have managed to even pass two years of higher education while smoking dope everyday.

So… The whole shebang becomes a bit of a hoohah, and then you think about Moses, and what he would do. This, of course, leads to the idea that instead of:

a) All going home to watch TV and sit in a nice centrally heated house, because 'of the revolution, man'. Or,

b) Actually leading the revolution.

You consider the possibility of staying in Glastonbury festival walking around the countryside for 40 years much like the Jews did during their Diaspora of Egypt in the desert, albeit with better scenery and more rock and roll. You then get a little paranoid, because:

LOVE IN THE PRISON OF PSYCHOSIS

a) You're stoned, and a 1,000 people are looking for guidance, and all you want is another joint and a cup of tea.

b) However much they like Glastonbury festival, a forty-year-long version might not go down all that well, however good your intentions.

c) At least the desert was sunny most of the time.

d) They'd soon run out of food, and, although you have always had a deep and profound belief in the Lord, it never quite stretched to the levels whereby manna from Heaven might literally fall out from the sky to feed the masses. Which leads to:

e) What would Jesus do? Feed the 5,000? Well, once again, you believe in the Lord almighty, but although someone on E has just mistaken you for the 'second coming' in the rave tent whilst watching the Chemical Brothers, you look at the plate of noodles in your hand, and the half eaten Donut, and, even though you're off your face on cannabis, not even that heady delight will stretch to the delusion that you could feed 5,000 people by creating the 'miracle of the noodles and Donuts'.

So, you get doubly paranoid, because although you're convinced the Lord loves you, which you have been told is the case on numerous occasions, your faith falters on the dichotomy between 'Faith in a tangible, fairly logical, 'higher dimension' kind of thing that seems totally plausible, even from a scientific point of view, while tripping', or 'Faith in a man with a beard who is creator of the universe who thinks you're such a righteous bloke, he will now give a load of free grub to this bunch of druggies because he really vibes with your idea of love and peace'.

This dichotomy of these two considerations then doubly splits into two more potential poles of associated extrapolation of 'what might be real', and then you realise you have no idea what 'reality' is anyway, because you've been high as a kite for half a decade, and have often mused on the very notion of what the fundamental basics of 'reality' actually are, and how it affects the mind, or how the mind effects the physical world, and...

And the mind has spiralled off on a tangent once again, in the middle of a field, when a rather strange looking hippy caked in mud, tattoos and piercings looks at you through his hideous facial forest with blazed eyes as though he's thinking 'My God, I look like Captain Caveman mixed with Robinson Crusoe, and a splash of Maori thrown in for good measure, and I've never been as off my tits as that guy, and he's clean shaven'. At which point you just think, 'well, I don't know that that is what he's thinking for sure, so why don't I ask him?'

So you approach the wild man of Glastonbury, who no doubt thinks Armageddon is definitely going to happen this year, even though he's thought that every year for twenty years, and say: "Care for a noodle, old boy?"

LOVE IN THE PRISON OF PSYCHOSIS

To which his wild eyes turn even wider... Wider than Rusty Lee's buttocks combined, and he runs into the crowd screaming:
"THE MAN'S A NUTTER!" as you ponder on what you've actually said that would generate such a reaction, and exactly what right does he have to call you a nutter when at least you've got a mildly attractive girlfriend and don't look like a barbaric psychopath with hair that reminds you of the yeti's crotch.
So you turn around, and a paper is thrown down at your feet, and your girlfriend, who's just grabbed the tall man's testicles who's standing slightly to the side and behind her thinking they were yours, begins to flick through them, red with embarrassment and hilarity that she's just felt up some stranger who walks off with a smile wide enough to destabilise both his cheekbones. She flicks through the paper, and leaves it on a page which simply says 'Break me Lex' next to a picture of a black king, and you have a massive moment where you connect everything that is going on around you to that one particular image, and think 'My GOD! They want me to paralyse the king!' And with complete disgust at the mission you think you've been given, you return back to the tent astonished at the coded brief, and thinking to yourself, 'I must not do what I think I might, or might not, have been told / commanded / suggested / authorised / pleaded / asked to do', due to the fact that it is probably some kind of conspiratorial subtle Illuminati Manchurian trigger, and you're not even sure if your right in the head

anyway, because there's a voice in your head saying: "Are you the golden lamb?"

Anyway... Enough about the razzle dazzle of a bygone mindbomb that occurred within the vicinity of about 100,000 unwilling volunteers (I scaled the fence for the second time. I don't pay to go to Satan's lair).

This evening, as I plotted my vengeance against 'the one who wronged the light', I decided I'd travel the spaghetti roads of my local (rather uninspiring) locus, seeking adventure.

Now... here is a case in point. When I use the term 'Adventure', I don't mean it in an Indiana Jones / James Bond sense, because I have a problem with killing and dealing with hardened criminals, given that the whole deal is an imaginative wet dream anyway. I have been known to have the finest adventures when sauntering down the cement tracks of my local globule of infrastructure and ogling the beautician who works at the hairdressers while munching on a bacon and cheese baguette and considering the finer aspects of a post-modern neo cruise into levels of ultimate potentiality that subjugate all given philosophies up unto this given time. Which is great, because although I only have a pathetic degree in theological fundamentals, I am also in the rather privileged position of knowing that the wanker who marked me down didn't know where my agenda was coming from, and, THEREFORE, his mother was a fat arse who smelt of poor odours.

LOVE IN THE PRISON OF PSYCHOSIS

Anyway, this is not the point. In the spirit of cutting edge literature, I will seek to inform you of the reality that I experienced this very evening. I drove in my U.R.C. Model 4 – the particle express, (A silver slice of perfect Teutonic engineering carved from the finest of minerals), to way point 'curdled babe', whereupon I sat, lonesome. (as is typical, due to a fine blend of eleven hurts and vices, the most typical of which is 'misogyny from an perspective of deep insight', mixed with a general misanthropic sneer at the temporal bollocks that mortals mentally masturbate over).

Do not think me an ill citizen, or a vagabond of the heart when I spill these raven terms. I simply mean to utter the fact that my generation, which I refer to now as Generation X-Tinct, (partly thanks to the fact that they all are weird, and talk drug fuelled bollocks), is on a major losing streak. Here is the evidence:

Pub 'curdled babe':

I drank a pint of Stella Artois on my own as I listened to two young women, one looking plain faced and angular, with what wouldn't pass for a wig in a shop as a true hairstyle discussing with this rather delicious feline the finer points of a well known current American drama. It was like listening to the 'society that Sodom wished it had been' as she unfurled one element of it's dramatic content after another, and, in a slightly heady mismatch of 'is this real, or is this delusional', I listened intently as she talked of the following:

Transvestites.

Serial killers who cut open girls mouths.

Adulterers who have skin grafts.

Tattooed homosexuals who slept with their best friend's girl.

A hero called Christian.

A kidnapping, involving a wedding marred in hatred.

Anal penetration by a doctor sporting dog tags.

As I left this Gemini of souls who were so engrossed in the finer points of a seriously sordid USA TV emission, I was forced to ask if I was right in thinking they were discussing a program, and that it wasn't the latest shenanigans in their personal life based within a small rural village community in the south of England.

Luckily, I was right... It was a program after all (The fevered imaginings of some psycho nut with a quill instead of knife, who'd slept his way into the foremost reaches of an American broadcast corporation and convinced the wide eyed slavering executives that a program so laced in decadence was what the world needed post September 11th). All that mattered was that the babe (and yay, verily I say unto thee, she was immaculate in a south of England random pub bird kind of Aphrodite way) played with her hair and laughed in glee as I attempted to curry my favour with the duo of allies.

So I left, and, streaming along the concrete rivulets, I made way to my second point of random inspection.

At this juncture, I would like to point out the weirdness I have between 'randomness', and 'so called freedom'. Daily diurnal passing of the machinations of a functional and maintained society obsessing with material wealth seems to be a miraculous event, if the evident reality of a sub-tribe of complete antagonism due to chronic psychosis wasn't increasing prevalent.

Nevermind... Tis a moot point, but the small focus on that collection of material data is nonetheless necessary due to the situation I see arising:

"People are stupid twats".

I will expand on this 'point' later, if you're lucky, due to the fact that although I seek freedom, if the freedom I sought ever manifested, only hell would endure. So... Betwixt this two parallel field of what is / isn't freedom, I plough my furrow continuously with a sceptical eye.

Anyway... Without wishing to bore you to duct water with the be all and end all of this particular spiral of my own particular element of what might or might not have been occurring psycho actively in one particular (and let's face it, possibly (or not possibly) very insignificant GPS location), I entered the 'second place'. A public domicile of some reverence within my native topography, as:

a) There was a bit of a 60's bass playing legend who owned it.
b) I fancied the pants off one of the barmaids (Who wasn't present this day in the year of our so called 'Lord').
c) It might show promise, as a meeting point for some fairly random cranium discharges should I feel so supercilious.

Alas... The half pint downed in this slim neck of the woods was not for celebrating en masse, and I will only go so far to say that aside from hearing the legislated factors revolving around 'private members clubs' from a man who was presumably half Orc, and the fact that a hero barman warned me not to question God… Little occurred.

So, punishing my vehicle into first, second, and then third and fourth, I set for home, not ceasing as the mellifluous tones of 'My culture' by One Giant Leap reverberated about my ears.

It was in my local, where, and I say this with a pinch of salt, or, at least, a modicum of sodium chloride, I usually embarrass myself by 'being totally individual'. (Rather than heeding the transient methods of a society founded on the basics), I indulged in a rather pleasing discourse with the young Great who works there. He believes wholeheartedly that he will be the next Prime Minister of Britain, and, even though he got a U in his A-Level politics, his vision remains undaunted. (Even though he has had the vote of over 300 people who in his psychohistory have agreed to mark the X upon the hotspot, and place him in overall control). Now… I got a D at A-Level politics, which made me paranoid and insecure for over half a decade thinking I was a complete shit for brains even though I never did the work, and yet this rather hirsute young upstart still thinks he's in with a running, which supposes to me that:

- a) He's smoked too much gear, which might be the case… BUT…
- b) So did I, but at least I didn't get a U. BUT…
- c) He stills believes he's smarter than everyone… BECAUSE

d) He reckons the person who marked him didn't know 'da shit'.

While we thus discussed the seven deadly sins, spending at least ten minutes trying to collate each 'deadly sin' because it's hard to officially recollect seven abstract psychological entities when you're both neither quite sure of what it is you're trying to remember, and attempting to memorise what is it you've already just said after a drink.

It was then that the major 'faux pas' was manifested however, and I glanced a deep insight into the methods of a teenager's pride.

Young Jane from work walked in, and, seeing as she'd rebutted my 'one time offer only, folks!' of going for a drink, even though her acne problem was so acute, she'd never sent a litre of blood to my groin in her presence, I could see she was a 'figure of some sexual focus' for the young Great, and her 'friend' (Some stud who'd pump her, but didn't want to know long term, because she was just a mere townie).

What she failed to appreciate, however, after I'd joked that I liked her Worzel Gummage hairdo, was that this 'stud' of hers... Who had gone to the same local prep school as this noxious scribe, always looked like a gunning loon to me, and that if she thought he was 'le chiens boules', then quite frankly... No wonder she was only seventeen. Because he was such a Sopwith camel of a flight plan, that I'd phantom his jet stream any day with A2A missiles and not give a shit what his deep agenda was, because he'd given away his whole *raison d'etre* to me in one gowning smile to the local drunkard, and that... Ladies and gentlemen... was enough in my book to have the man forever labelled a 'TOSSER'.

Perhaps I am being a little too harsh. I suspect his parents love him, much in the same way my mother loves me, even though I'm clinically psychotic.

So I'm in the shop again... This little cell like an ineffective money drip, waiting, pontificating, listening, in order to earn beer and cigarette tokens. A huge man is trying to be nice to me. I'm worried he's a psycho gimp, and wants to rape me. He's speaking to me as I write this, but luckily he can't see the screen. I sense a sadness about him, as though his corpulence and bizarre facial hair has failed to garner him the dames he secretly masturbates over in his lair ridden with posters of models he'll never manage to score with. Bibles too... Possibly. Loads of them. Crucifixes above his soiled mattress. I bet he prays to Jesus nightly hoping for an escape from that bulky frame, and to have the agile and taught Spiderman like body I sport. But then, I don't get the girls either. Because I have a look in my eye that says 'stay away, I've been hurt too much', and a grin that suffixes that hostile vision with 'And I'm over it, and I now just see women as sex objects. A label you created for yourself by your actions'.

'Hey Dude' by Kula Shaker comes on the stereo, and as I'm punching these digits right on the edge of time's humungous onslaught of experience, the massive man leaves with a comment designed to be friendly, and I smile happily to see him go, thinking 'Perhaps he is really my best friend?'

Not only that, but we had two fairly cracking looking girls in here before. Both very slim... Too slim in fact... Beanpoles... But possessing a definite desirability. I talked to them about films, and felt my monotone 'posh' drawl cough and splutter in their presence as I tried to impress them by not trying to impress them... Which completely failed to impress them. These girls are kind of posh too. People sometimes think the posh say 'the rain in Spain falls mainly on the plain', but the REALLY distinguished actually say: "The on-going pluvial precipitation situation transpires generally in *la region de Espana*" – 'cos we speak well good, *innit?*

I know people they speak of, in their enthusiasm, and I consider their high spiritedness... Because they are either:

a) Generally bubbly women.

b) Bubbly because they quite like me.

c) Bubbly because their boyfriends are great in the sack, and they know I'm a crap lay, and want to taunt me surreptitiously. Or,

d) They're on cocaine.

The reality could go either way, but I manage to get them to hire 'the 40 year old virgin', which I happen to think is a lovely little comedy about love and sex.

They leave, and are replaced with a mother and her three children. It is only when I am waiting for them to decide on which computer game to buy, and I suddenly think 'Christ, I'm masturbating too much at home', that I thank the Lord that telepathy is probably not possible. Now, you might consider me an Onanist... But I'll have you know I had sex before I had an orgasm. That isn't saying much. I didn't have an orgasm until the age of 17. I didn't even know what was meant to happen, and I went to a private school for Goodness sake. I remember coming back to my study to go to bed stoned, and thinking 'I am going to wank until something happens that is possibly what all my friends talk about, and I'm not going to stop unless I pass out through physically exhaustion, or the damn thing comes off in my hand'.

So I did...

I throttled my member for ages, in a state of heightened arousal, and I did not quit on my mission, even though I was crying out with boredom and fear that I was sexually defunct... and then... THEN... Finally, at the age of 17, I felt that muscular all over body sensation of 'power surge', and made a mess of my duvet. Still... It was worth it... It proved I was virile and potent, and I could finally know what it was that teenage boys spent hours exhilarating over. Still, I felt like a pervert... But then... I wasn't alone. There were millions of us.

(At this juncture, I would like to point out that I do not believe Onanism is a mortal sin. I believe it is a completely natural outlet of desire, and healthy even, so that people don't walk around frenzied and uptight and liable to jump on poor innocent women through sheer frustration). The idea that

LOVE IN THE PRISON OF PSYCHOSIS

God made women desirable, and yet we are not meant to experience these sensations of sexuality is absurd. Ok, so the 144,000 who are saved come the Apocalypse may all be virgins... But I'd be jolly well interested to find out how they were made in the first place... What a stupid idea).

I pop out for a cigarette, and have that strong feeling that I want to visit India before I die. I am sick of being located in the same GPS point for so much time... It's boring, as though humans have to be stationed in their zones as part of the grand pyramid of power. I want more fluidity, more free roaming, and less hostile looks from people who think they know a damn thing. One of the best reasons for studying philosophy is that not only do you realise that the greatest minds who ever lived didn't actually know what was going on, but you learn how to realise that no one knows what is going on in a very intelligent way. Which is marvellous, because that means you can basically think what you like, and with a few clever sentences, be considered a genius because you've read the bible on LSD, got a degree while schizophrenic, and NO ONE has the right to mess with you... Because yes... It IS big, it IS clever, and it's also slightly disturbing.

I've met Stalinists working in my local restaurant. Meglomaniacs in my local pub. Physicians in the Co-op. Murderers who are now lawyers. Prussian descendants of the royal family working in a tile shop. Neo Nazi's in retirement towns. It's madness... Madness I say, and surely the accusation of me as psychotic is based on no given evidence other than I expect more out of life than I should.

Let us deconstruct my 'insanity' to see if it really stands up to the notion. What is madness? Is 'anger' madness? A lot of people are angry... I'm rarely angry. I'm quite happy a lot of the time, but that's because I've been blessed from on high by a divine force. Now... It's when I say stuff like this that people start to think I'm crazy. And herein lies the rub. For what I am saying is TOTAL TRUTH. Maybe in the future, people will know what I'm riffling about. It's illumination... The apotheosis of potential consciousness, and I reached the Everest of insight. This proved to me a few fundamental TRUTHS:

1) There is more to being a human than merely being a slightly smarter animal with an opposable thumb.
2) There IS a higher power... Or divine force... Or 'something' that operates at a subtle level of far, far deeper intelligence than mere mortals can access.
3) I am completely lucky to know about this.
4) Most people don't have a clue what I'm on about.
5) It's the true origin of the artistic depiction of halos, and not, as Dan Brown and other Pagan's would have it, an ancient pagan sun worship thing.
6) Gold is the colour of enlightenment.

LOVE IN THE PRISON OF PSYCHOSIS

With these 6 FACTS... I soar through the matrix like a slightly more grounded Neo merely guessing at what I'm now meant to do with the given evidence. Sure... It's great for me... But notice how ironic the 'evidence many seek of there being more' is generated. It lies within the mind... And can others see into that mind? No... So, in inner space, I am totally utopian, and protected from all evils by a miraculous event of heavenly wonder... But the outside, physical world? They still are unaware of my spiritual event. So, I take to the computer, and I write, and I write, and I write some more, desperately seeking to impart this most valuable knowledge.

After a momentary sojourn into the likelihood of how much I comprehend existence compared to that of the butcher next door, or the monstrosity of a woman at the local library, I realise how Nelson Mandela has ruled. He just danced in public, and said positive things... That is so EASY!!! What a cop out... I could do that. It's basically the 'dancing and singing 'think happy thoughts' agenda'.

Man... We've been robbed. No wonder he's so praised. It's like having a black Tellytubby in charge of a bunch of confused people. What an intelligent solution. Perhaps Britain should do it. Maybe everyone in the 'Psychedelic party' (a political movement I am thinking of founding), should simply stand in the halls of Parliament grooving to the beat and saying cool things, like:

"Peace for all, always..."

"Money is only measured by how desperate to drive a Mercedes you are, and live in a house with more bedrooms than you'll ever need."

"We all bleed red."

"Cheryl from 'Girls aloud' is da bomb!"

"Let's turn the next election into a reality TV show called 'Prime Minister Idol', or do one for the new royal family called 'The Rex Factor".

"Steve Martin for President!"

People are so weird. I was just watching the world pass by outside, and a chap smiles at me and says 'Afternoon'. Of course, you might not see this as particularly weird, but basically, he's just walked passed me, smiled, and said 'Its post lunch time'. Or, if you will, it's like you walking passed someone you don't really know, and saying '2:49pm!'

And??? I know what the fecking time is... Can't you see I'm wearing a cheap but highly efficient Casio timepiece? Why don't you give me some valuable information? Something that can improve my life? Something like, "Would you like a free joint?"

Ok, now I've really done it.

I sauntered over to a massive truck delivering meat and surveyed the dead animals strung up on the inside.

"My God... It's a good thing I'm not a vegetarian," I said.

The man grunted something with a laconic smile, possibly wondering who on earth I was.

LOVE IN THE PRISON OF PSYCHOSIS

"I… I just wanted to see corpses," I said, and then walked off giggling, mentally kicking myself at saying something so utterly bizarre. He must now think I'm a right weirdo, but the site of dead pigs strung up by their rear trotters will probably stay with me for life. I knew a barman once who said he had two friends who used to work in an abattoir, and smash up pig brains when tripping on acid for 'fun'.

And *I'm* the one seeing a psychiatrist?

So many elements comprise an existence, and yet we cling to solution of money abating our paranoia… And to some extent, it does appease the general material confines of a world judged by physical value, but having just been given an I-pod for my birthday, I can safely say that some things are worth buying. What an incredibly wondrous invention (Designed by a Brit, I'll have you know). It only cost £200, and can hold over 7,000 of my favourite songs. I'm not even sure if I *have* 7,000 favourite songs, but I've download 435 songs so far, and I can select any one to play at any time with minimal fuss. It's absolutely excellent, and I advise all 'techno-legends' to buy one… It is quality personnel equipment.

Not only that, but the day is brimming with good news for me. My film that I wrote and directed a few years ago is going to be played in 200 Spanish cinema's, and an ideas capture manager is possibly interested in discussing my latest idea for a mobile phones company. Furthermore, I have a cunning plan for a website, and my silly short film I made for free about a triad of ninjas making tea completely by myself one bored Sunday (playing all three ninjas) is being downloaded on the Internet by about 200 people a day. Also, He-man is speaking to me for advice on a number of website issues, and I have a lady who once me to make a music video for her son.

The icing on the cake, however, has to be that a young girl whose friends and mother I join for 'quiz night' informed me just now that they won last night. They only won by three points mind you, and I answered at least four questions for them, which just goes to show... I can help people in 'pub quiz' need.

So... As the shimmering of time gleams it's crypto-messaging at me in a variety of bizarre new ways, I take all thoughts of desiring to place a bullet in the head of the 'monkey boned jizz boy' melt into a distant foolish memory. Even as the ultimate assassin, one death generated by my livid trigger finger would shine forever a decadent, showery residue of venom in an otherwise halcyon kaleidoscopic mind of positive sensations, and cling to my fevered being as a terrible malediction of decision. I doubt in my mind he'll be as blessed with the craved experience I know and foster, and should we meet again in this labyrinth of molecular reality, like before, I'll terrify him with just a knowing look – such is the illicit majesty of his punkdom crappery.

LOVE IN THE PRISON OF PSYCHOSIS

Thus... Although I have not won the palm and digits of the fair Danni, I settle into a new supposed spiral of events that might leave of erroneous history of misdemeanours, and trundle off further into the futures sprawling cornucopia of mysteries. I might try to win an affectionate look from Danni sometime in that path, and know that she might be too tender of reason to garner the flow of my soul atop her marble frame, but we may dwell within a vicinity bonded through at least one element of affection, rather than rust and spasm in the terrible catacombs of a complex location built on animosity.

The prison walls break free for a moment, and I am reminded in the affectionate eyes of a new customer that indeed, life's elements are comprised of many strange and random events, and to try and quantify all of that myriad of data into one tome that dispels one iota of deeper comprehension is simply one tiny dot in the cerebral social mosaic of civilisation.

Thus like a letter to an ancient church, I rescind all methods of pernicious thinking I have indulged in up until now, and repent daily, although unable to stop my desire to get high, and think of time now as a gift... As every minute one is still alive and innocent is laced with nothing but hope in a world of simple mortals and sinners. I realise that the betrayal of my first love, and the desire to be with Danni are just two love triangles I've been a part of with me at a different angle in each scenario, and I should employ 'psychological meditation on alternate perspectives' in order to cope with the traces of hurt that linger in my chronology. Yet, like Jamelia sings in 'thank you', 'for every last bruise you gave me, for every time you made my cry, I thank you, because now I'm stronger'.

It's pretty deep stuff... and moulded about a beautiful pop ballad.

Anyway... Enough is enough of this prevarication with textual exploits... I must work on Project 2 – The intrazone, if only so the foul punishments of pagan scummers don't unfurl decadent reprisal for merely independent thinking.

White hoodie, black combats, and a T-shirt with Latin sported, I take my trusty I-Pod and other five necessary street artefacts, including my kid's sunglasses, (bought because they look like silver cyborg fun), and saunter into the future knowing that 'doing good' eventually generates a unique personal existence of some relevance in an increasingly paranoid world.